The detail of the analysis is excellent and, whilst not always easy, . . . it is for the most part written in plain English. This is a welcome change from the elaborate prose of so many American community texts . . . . Good use is made of the wealth of published community work case studies to illustrate each step in the work process.

The book will be a God-send to community work teachers who, like their social work colleagues, are for the most part trying to teach a craft they no longer practise themselves from within an academic institution, divorced from the reality of that practice. It is a good combination of intellectual rigour applied to practical knowledge.

British Journal of Social Work

will be widely read and used for training purposes. The book is certainly geared to the training of the neighbourhood worker as neighbourhood work has typically been organised and practised over the past decade or so.

Critical Social Policy

a solid and substantial text on locality-based organizing and one of the most outstanding works on the subject available. Henderson and Thomas synthesize a wealth of literature from the United Kingdom and the United States, using a framework that is well suited to their subject. The American material, which tends to be more theoretical, is brought alive when integrated with the substantial body of case studies and theoretical work done in the United Kindom over the last twenty-five years.

Social Work (USA)

SKILLS IN
NEIGHBOURHOOD WORK

SKILLS IN NEIGHBOURHOOD WORK

Paul Henderson
David N. Thomas

National Institute for Social Work

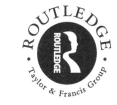

London and New York

First published 1980 by Unwin Hyman Ltd
Second edition 1987
Fourth impression 1990

Reprinted 1992, 1994, 1996, 2000
by Routledge
11 New Fetter Lane, London EC4P 4EE

Simultaneously published in the USA and Canada
by Routledge
29 West 35th Street, New York, NY 10001

Routledge is an imprint of the Taylor & Francis Group

Typeset in Times by Columns Design and
Production Services Ltd, Reading
Printed and bound in Great Britain by
Biddles Ltd, www.Biddles.co.uk

British Library Cataloguing in Publication Data
A catalogue record for this book is available from the British Library

Library of Congress Cataloguing in Publication Data
A catalogue record for this book is available from the Library of Congress

ISBN 0–415–08393–1

For our children
   Juliet, Jamie and Barnaby
   Danny and Siân

Contents

CONTENTS

Two video tapes have been made to be used with this book. Information about these tapes can be found at the back of the book, together with details of other publications about working in neighbourhoods.

The National Institute for Social Work offers a range of training, research and consultancy services about community development and community-based social work. For information on these, please telephone:

David Thomas on 01 387 9681 or Paul Henderson at the Institute's northern office in Leeds − 0532 798250.

Acknowledgements

The writing of this book has been achieved through a good deal of collaboration with many people in different parts of the country. We could not have produced it without the help of Jacki Reason who has been a continuing source of patience, support and hard work in this and other projects.

We owe a considerable debt to those practitioners to whom we have been consultants and to those who attended our workshops on neighbourhood work skills. This book originated from discussions in those sessions. We developed the contents of specific chapters in seminars with students on the National Institute's three-month course – in particular Ted Duckett, Margaret Malcolm, Don Sandford, Joyce Mosely, Colin Barnes, Vernon Tudor and Kevin Loughran in Belfast. Our ideas were then rigorously reviewed with Sarah del Tufo and Chris Warren, who may not be aware of how important their encouragement was to us.

The people mentioned above were not only students; they were, and still are, practitioners. We obtained more views from practitioners by sending the first draft of the book to a number of community workers, and we are extremely grateful for the extensive comments and suggestions made by Clem and Felicity McCartney in Northern Ireland, Chris Dean and Joan Munro. They helped us, at a crucial stage, to revise what we had written, making it more relevant to the interests of practitioners.

A second draft was produced, and we thought it essential to find out how useful it would be to trainers and students in community work. We approached some trainers who agreed to read it from this point of view and their advice had considerable impact on the way in which we ordered and presented our material. It is with respect that we express our gratitude to these trainers: Phil Bryers in Scotland, Ann Curno, John Haines, David Jones and Laurence Tasker, as well as Han Hidalgo and Jacques van Berkel of the University of Tilburg, Holland.

All these people helped to make this book possible; there are a greater number, however, who made it necessary, and they are the neighbourhood workers who seek to help local residents win resources, power and self-respect. We hope that what we have written will help them and local people in their work. Although our debt to individuals is deep and widespread, the responsibility for this book's content and any shortcomings rests with us.

The Second Edition

This second edition was made possible by grants from the Wates and Baring Foundations, and we are grateful for their support. We were helped in preparing it by Bill Bourne, Ruth Page and Stevie Krayer, and by a number of practitioners and trainers who responded to our request for help in revising the book. Our thanks, also, to Ad Raspe of the Netherlands Institute for Community Development whose enterprise and hard work led to the Dutch translation of the book; and to Alex Meigh and Chris Andrews of 3/4" Productions who helped in making the videotape, *Learning About Community Work*, that derives from parts of this book. Finally, we are grateful to *Community Care* for allowing us to use some material first published by them on 1 August 1985.

Introduction

We have written this book to help those working in neighbour-hoods. It is intended both for people who do neighbourhood work as a full-time job, and also for those who put into practice its principles and methods as part of another profession, such as social work or youth work. We hope it will be of use to anyone who wishes to develop groups, networks and linkages in a neighbourhood, and to help local people tackle needs and issues that affect their livelihood.

This group of potential readers comprises most of those identified in a report from the Gulbenkian Foundation (1984):

- people working full- or part-time as community workers. According to a national survey carried out by Francis *et al.* (1984) there are some 5,500 such workers in the United Kingdom, the large majority of whom are in the voluntary sector;
- staff whose major function is not necessarily to do neighbour-hood work, but who draw upon it as a method, and whose agencies are intimately associated with community affairs and issues. Examples are the staff of community relations commit-tees, and of councils of voluntary service; and welfare rights officers, intermediate treatment workers, community artists, community tutors and those in legal, housing, consumer, and general advice centres;
- workers and students in welfare, health and related fields who want to assimilate the insights and methods of neighbourhood work in order better to carry out their own primary tasks. There is an increasing number of such staff in medicine, education, social work, planning, the youth service, and the probation service. We try to indicate, towards the end of this introduction, how this book might be useful to those involved in community social work, and to workers who have begun to operate from neighbourhood projects and family centres;

1

- the staff, volunteer workers and members of both local and regional self-help groups;
- local residents involved in a wide variety of neighbourhood groups and activities;
- the clergy and congregations of the churches, particularly those in the kinds of urban priority areas analysed in the Archbishop of Canterbury's Commission (1985). Case studies of church based neighbourhood work have been published by the British Council of Churches (see Godfrey, 1985).

When the first edition of this book was published in 1980, it was one of the few texts available to help practitioners and students be more effective neighbourhood workers. That is no longer the case; there have been a number of further British contributions to the practice theory of neighbourhood work including the 1982 books of Twelvetrees and the Bryants. Also available are a number of practical handbooks, such as Gibson's and that of Richardson on self-help groups, both published in 1984. Indeed, there has been a plethora of 'how-to-do-it' books; some of the best of these are reviewed in the October issues of the *Community Development Journal* in 1984 and 1985 with full details of the content and how to obtain them.

The publication of books dealing with issues in community work has also carried on apace. For example, since 1980 the Association of Community Workers has published books on racism, the state, and participation. There have also been case studies of particular projects, for example those by Henderson *et al.* (1983) and Taylor (1983). In addition, today's reader has access to research publications about community work: Francis's survey (1984) of community workers tells us how many there are, who employs them, as well as information about their age, sex, ethnicity, training and salary. The research report from Davies and Crousaz (1982) provides data on what community workers do with their time, and the constraints and opportunities that they face in employment.

Finally, there have been a number of reviews of community work, including the two published by Thomas in 1983 that look at the history, practice, training and research of community work in the United Kingdom. A complementary view is provided in the book on community work and the state edited by Craig (1982).

It is self-evident that this recent literature has its roots in British community work practice. But an interesting change has taken place since the late 1970s: the practice of neighbourhood work is now less influenced by United States programmes and publications. There has been more attention paid to experiences in mainland Europe. This is reflected, for example, in the Dutch seminars and exchanges organised by the Federation of Community Work Training Groups, and in the work of the European Community Development Exchange.

It has to be noted, too, that the Dutch experience has had some influence on discussions about the role of a national resource centre, and its relationship to regional structures for the support of neighbourhood workers and local activists. The working party established by the Gulbenkian Foundation identified a consensus in favour of a national centre; consultations still in progress at the beginning of 1986 indicate an interest in the 'Dutch model' that combines a national centre with other resources strategically located in regional agencies and networks.

And practice itself has changed. It has been shaped by swingeing cuts in housing, health, education and income maintenance programmes, by rising levels of unemployment and by the general malaise that has afflicted the British economy. Neighbourhood workers are finding it harder to organise and motivate people, particularly in the neighbourhoods of the inner city. Local authorities have fewer resources to compete for, residents are pessimistic about the efficacy of collective action, their optimism about themselves and the future dampened by unemployment and by the refusal of government to pay attention to the unhappiness and deprivation which its management of the economy has helped to bring about. Cleavages between young and old, black and white, and those in and out of work seem to bode ill for the neighbourhood worker who seeks to bring people together to achieve some improvement in their well-being. Urban residents seem to prefer staying at home rather than taking part in community activities, protected by multiple locks and alsation dogs, suspicious of each other, and fearful of crime and harassment.

Some of these factors have brought about a change in what neighbourhood workers do. There is, for example, greater interest today in schemes related to economic development and job creation; there is more concern with 'specialist' rather than 'generalist' neighbourhood work, with both management committees and workers preferring to work on particular issues in particular fields – in health, education and employment creation, for instance.

The Importance of the Neighbourhood

It is becoming equally apparent that more and more people are having to spend more and more time at home and in their neighbourhood. This is occurring because of:

- unemployment, early retirement, job-sharing and other changes in the patterns of work;
- demographic changes such as the proportion of older people in the population;
- policy changes such as the removal of people from institutions to care in the community.

The scarcity and cost of transport and energy may help to keep people more 'local' than they have been in the past; and some trends in new technological developments seem to have a 'localising' effect. For example, there is the prospect of office workers being able to work at home and at company-owned neighbourhood offices. The social and political consequences of this trend towards localism has been discussed elsewhere by one of the authors (see Thomas, 1986).

For the neighbourhood worker, there are two major issues to consider. First, many of the neighbourhoods in which people are spending more of their time are materially in a state of disrepair. Second, the social fabric of these neighbourhoods is in no less a state of neglect: not only are people set apart from each other by conflicts and scapegoating, but we may wonder whether people know *how* to manage their relationships with each other. This state of affairs may have come about partly because social skills involved in neighbouring and networking may have atrophied over a period in which people enjoyed a private, home-centred life that was combined with the pursuit of work and leisure in areas outside the neighbourhood. A consequence is that many people find themselves for much of their day in a neighbourhood, but not of it.

The 'localisation' of everyday life has been paralleled by trends towards the localisation of services provided both by local government departments and large voluntary organisations. A number of professions, most notably social work, have discovered the neighbourhood as a base for delivering services and as a potential resource in the development of care. Several local authorities have moved towards the decentralisation of 'town hall' functions, and both socialist and conservative politicians have, for different purposes and values, committed themselves to various forms of community care and self-help, and to a range of co-operative or consumer-led enterprises.

The Poverty of Neighbourhood Theory

It has been a paradox of British neighbourhood work that its practitioners or trainers have done little to develop ideas about the neighbourhood. They have generally given more attention to devising and using theories about things other than the local – about the state or about class, for example. Neighbourhood work has also been characterised by a fetish with the vertical, with what has been called 'smash-and-grab' community work. Much theory and discussion has centred on the vertical relationships between community groups and resource holders, and on the means by which such groups can grab the resources they need. This concern with community action has rarely been matched by an interest in community interaction, and the relationship between the two has not attracted much intellectual or practical attention. So there is in neighbourhood work, even today, a poverty of theorising about the horizontal, about networks and linkages, roles and responsibilities, and the extent and quality of people's interactions with one another.

It has to be said, too, that social policy in the United Kingdom has had a *laissez-faire* attitude to the development of communities. The neighbourhood has been seen as the environment or framework within which other social systems operate; rarely has the neighbourhood been seen as a unit in its own right, as an important element of social structure, about which it is proper to ask evaluative questions about its functioning and state of repair.

What we particularly lack is a *generic* theory of the neighbourhood and neighbourhood work. By this we mean a theory that makes sense to, and is usable by, a whole range of practitioners interested in the neighbourhood – community workers, social workers, job creation experts, health workers, and so on. We suggest that such a generic theory is provided by the idea of 'community capability', which we shall describe below. This idea is generic because not only is capability at the heart of the specific goals of particular neighbourhood groups, but it is a quality or an attribute whose presence is essential if, for example, schemes to provide community care are to be successful. Creating communities that are capable, *if the right resources are at their disposal*, to manage their own internal relations and responsibilities, and to deal with power and resource holders outside the neighbourhood, is an implicit goal of much neighbourhood work and decentralised forms of local government and voluntary sector provisions.

Defining Community Capability

The idea of community capability is taken from the research of Wallman (1982), Schoenberg (1979) and Schoenberg and Rosenbaum (1980) who have explored the concept of viability in local communities, and the way residents pursue their livelihood.

There lies behind these particular meanings of community capacity a wider general notion, defined by Schoenberg in the following way:

> A capable or viable community is one in which its residents work together to influence various aspects of the local social order, in which residents set goals for collective life, and in which they have the ability to carry out work to accomplish these goals.

Following, but building upon Schoenberg's work, we would say that a locality achieves this kind of capability if it can:

– establish mechanisms to define and enforce shared agreements about public roles and responsibilities. These would vary from neighbourhood to neighbourhood but would certainly include

agreements about personal safety, the identification of strangers, the maintenance of common property, the disposal of rubbish and the behaviour of children;
- set up both formal and informal organisations in the locality which provide for communication, the identification of leadership, the learning of skills, and the ability to define, and to take action upon, the various interests of the neighbourhood to those outside it;
- make inputs on policy and political decision-making that affects the neighbourhood;
- maintain linkages to public and private resource holders;
- establish mechanisms, formal and informal, through which exchanges are created between conflicting interests, needs and groups in the neighbourhood.

There are a number of points to be made about community capability: in most working-class neighbourhoods these kinds of mechanisms and organisation will not be created or sustained without the skilled intervention of neighbourhood workers, and the provision of basic administrative and servicing resources.

The challenge faced by professionals in fields such as housing, health, social work and education is to realise that they must seek not just to deliver services to meet people's needs but to do so in a way that enhances people's autonomy, self-respect and their ability to work together to solve common problems. At the heart of the development of capable communities is the understanding that the *way* in which they carry out their professional role – that is, the neighbourhood-sensitive way in which they carry it out – is as important as the meeting of needs that individuals bring to them.

As far as neighbourhood workers are concerned, they cannot do very much until they begin to see themselves – and to be so recognised by politicians and policy makers – as instruments of the development of communities as capable social systems, rather than agents of particular groups in the community with a specific but limited task. Clearly, the creation and support of such action groups is essential to collective problem solving but they need to be seen only as a part of the development of the interacting community. Neighbourhood workers and policy makers need to develop their understanding, and skills in promoting, horizontal integration at the locality level. Their job is not only to help local people establish the kinds of organisations and networks identified by Schoenberg as necessary for community capability, but also to support people's participation in them, to make them work, to take up membership in groups, and to make efforts to sustain information and communication patterns.

A Special Word to Social Workers (and some others)

This section is written for social workers wishing to borrow ideas from neighbourhood work in order to do community social work. However, we believe the material in this section will also be useful to youth workers and education staff who are trying to explore the meaning of 'community youth work' and 'community education'. For such workers, they must adapt the ideas in the next few pages to their own circumstances: for community social work, read community youth work.

The advent of community social work has meant that more and more social services staff are having to dip a toe into the community, and to take the plunge into various forms of neighbourhood-based work. And for many, it has been a sink or swim experience, that has often created confusion about direction and method.

Community social work is about better meeting the needs of individuals and families. It is not neighbourhood work (helping groups organise and take action for the benefit of a wider constituency) but it is *in* the neighbourhood, and it *does* involve working with all kinds of groups and organisations. For this reason, community social work must borrow and adapt some of the methods of neighbourhood work, and that is why this book will be of value to social workers and other professionals wanting to intervene at the neighbourhood level.

Community social work is a team and agency strategy that comprises:

(1) a local role and site in a neighbourhood;
(2) a method that seeks to create a variety of networks and groups in a community, and, through doing so, developing new roles and responsibilities for people that are satisfying to themselves and of service to others;

8

(3) a new relationship between professional workers and local residents. In our opinion it is the development of this new kind of relationship that is at the heart of community social work, and provides the most testing, long-term challenge to those wishing to implement a strategy of community social work.

The Barclay Report (1982) came close to defining this relationship in its concept of partnership. Our definition of this principle of community social work is as follows:

Community social work is being created when what social workers are doing in a neighbourhood is done with the knowledge (though not always the consent) of people who live there; and that the basis of welfare policy and practice are known about and subject to open discussion and revision.

The development of this kind of relationship will depend on far greater openness and trust between professionals and non-professionals than usually exists today.

It means social workers being much better at demonstrating what they are doing, de-mystifying the tricks of the trade. It also requires them to be better at asking questions: 'How do you think services should be delivered here?' 'What kind of social work support or resources should be delivered here?' 'What kind of social work support or resources do you think this area needs?'

We come now to a seeming paradox in community social work. It is primarily concerned with improving services in response to the needs of individuals and families. Thus community social work is not something which is 'added on' to existing practice. Rather, it becomes the springboard from which social work plans its intervention, including statutory work.

Although it is a strategy better to meet the needs of individuals and families, it is also essential for social workers to develop a far more active perspective on community. Community social work is not just about recognising the community context, the backdrop against which social workers carry out their tasks. Communities have lives of their own. They are complex and full of conflicts. Social workers have to recognise this, not keep it at a distance with a passing nod of recognition. Some of the most useful writing on community available to social workers has come out of the

Church of England Children's Society projects; readers are recommended to refer to, for example, the texts by Holman (1983) and Adamson and Warren (1983).

Community Social Work: the Four C's

We have found it useful to describe community social work in terms of 'the four C's':

(1) practice capability;
(2) community capability;
(3) team capability;
(4) management capability.

   We will briefly say a little about each of these, in order to make it clear that community social work is not something that only the individual social worker does in the neighbourhood.

Practice Capability

In working in a neighbourhood, the social work team needs to ensure that its practice is capable of containing the following ingredients. We see these principles as being fundamental in determining strategies in community social work.

   Felt and expressed need, or really listening to what local people and consumers are saying and acting upon it. Taking this principle seriously poses a challenge to social work and demands radical changes in day-to-day practice. It is not the case that good social work has always adhered to this principle.

   Informal networks. This is a major element of community social work that was emphasised in the Barclay report but there are a number of difficulties; for example, the ease with which professionalised, large-scale welfare agencies can colonise informal networks, which by definition are fragile and loose-knit. Working with informal networks is fundamental to community social work, though applying this principle often exposes the deficiency in social work teams of their knowledge of community resources.

   Participation. Involving clients and local people in decisions about priorities and how services are delivered would seem to be axiomatic to community social work. Either social work seeks to engage with the community or it does not, and if it does it has to deliberately open its doors: put its goods on display, encourage response and debate, begin to share power. Relying upon local government representation, crucial though that is, requires parallel, complementary structures to facilitate such changes.

Agency development and co-ordination. At first sight, this may seem less challenging than the first three principles; but it is a mode of operation which should not be treated in an administrative sense, or seen as necessary only in order to achieve a specific task. It is often spoken of in defensive terms, whereas we visualise it as an active, and creative approach and one to be employed at all levels of an organisation. We are referring to development within an agency and also to co-ordination with other agencies, although clearly each will demand different approaches.

The *strategic* importance of a team's or a department's services, particularly the more effective integration of casework, groupwork and community work within a neighbourhood.

Awareness of the social work team as part of a neighbourhood system. This spells the end of the siege mentality that surrounds many social work offices. Part of this is the recognition of the users of social services as part of wider systems in and outside the neighbourhood. It goes hand in hand with developing a realistic picture of the users of the team's services.

We need to go beyond seeing people as resources to an appreciation of a person's wide range of needs – not just for specific social work services, but also those to do with home, educational and developmental matters. There is an implication here that community social work teams will include staff other than social workers (an adult educator, for example) and, second, that there will be a much more effective use of experts and resources in other departments and voluntary agencies.

Localisation of the team. This may mean the opening of patch offices; or attachments to schools and GP clinics; or the employment of more indigenous workers; or more staff living in the area in which they work; or team offices being available for a wide range of neighbourhood activities.

It will mean less use of the car, more informal contact with residents and the more conscious use of neighbourhood facilities, such as shopping and pubs, that allows for a greater degree of overlapping roles for social workers. What is certain is that localisation means far more than simply going patch.

Helping users and others in the community to take up more responsibility for neighbourhood functions such as socialisation, social control and mutual support, and achieving the resources to do this. In saying this, we are aware of the degree of change and reconceptualisation that will be required.

Recognising the *indivisibility* of need in a community; community social work is not about being confined to what is often described as 'social work issues'. On the contrary, it recognises that interweaving of need across the artificial boundaries of departments and social policies, and is thus able to respond (in the way described in the Seebohm report (HMSO, 1968)) to a range of need and issues in a neighbourhood.

Taken together these principles should indicate the fundamental change in direction that we assume for community social work.

Community Capability

We have already discussed this idea. If policy initiatives to establish community care or to use community resources are to be successful, then policy makers must understand the concept of community capability which such initiatives assume, and direct to it appropriate theoretical attention and practical resources. As for practitioners, part of their work in the neighbourhood will be to set up and support some of the organisations and networks as identified earlier that help it to be capable in its dealings with those outside, and in handling internal difficulties and issues.

In addition, there are three kinds of contributions to be made by the social worker in developing the interacting community:

(1) helping people to know about each other, and developing the concern and interest they take in what is happening to people in the community around them, being responsible for what goes on around them, and seeing the ways in which it is possible for residents to empathise with the fortunes and tribulations of their neighbours;
(2) identifying the different possibilities for role development and expansion in a locality, the opportunities for residents to take up roles (neighbour, volunteer, party activist, association

secretary, PTA member and so forth) that are satisfying to themselves and of service to others, and which, in turn, strengthen networks and contribute to people's knowledge of, and interest in, each other;

(3) working to ensure that both local people and other professionals recognise the significance of social resources (trust, information, identity, a sense of mattering, etc.) in the pursuit of livelihood.

Team Capability

Maintaining the complex integration and balance between the individual and the community is often at the centre of the intellectual and emotional exhaustion that characterises many social workers faced with implementing a strategy of community social work. But the difficulties are compounded by the need to understand the social work *team* as the third variable to be handled together with those of the individual and the community.

Community social work is thus not something done by the individual practitioner. It is a team strategy with far-reaching implications for the structure and procedures of the whole of a social services agency. Part of the flawed response of many councillors and senior managers to community social work is the assumption that it is only the basic grade worker whose practice and ideas have to change.

Community social work implies a *strong* concept of team work. By 'strong' we mean a portfolio of tasks and skills held by a team, with the team taking collective responsibility for the work being done by each of its members.

At one level, team members would generally need to be highly interactive. From our observations of community social work teams, this often takes the form of high morale, either because a team has had to stand firm together during a process of change and in the face of external scepticism, or because work satisfaction is high as a result of people learning about new ways of working, and being creative.

At another level, community social work teams have to be extremely good at planning and managing their work. A paradox of community social work is that more team autonomy and decentralisation, far from pointing individuals in the direction of libertarianism and unfettered freedom, demand tight team organisation and a deliberate attempt to design programmes of individual work, the sum of which make up a team-agreed whole. Clear objectives, determination to carry through identified priorities become all-important. So too does regular evaluation of programmes.

Inevitably, perhaps, the team leader's role in this way of working becomes critical. He or she has not only to be adept at encouraging and enabling colleagues but also skilled at being the pivot between the team and the rest of the agency. Carrying out both enabling and management functions demands an unusual combination of human qualities, skills, energy, and commitment. The active training and support required by team leaders should never be underestimated.

Management Capability

Expectations of the team leader role give us the clue to another evident feature of community social work; the community-based fieldwork team can never lose sight of the agency focus of its work. It should always be interested in drawing the entire agency into discussions and decisions about community social work.

Any idea that community social work is something that is only the province of fieldwork teams needs to be smartly disposed of. Community social work is an entirely different way of working, not merely change at the margins, and must be agency-wide. This is particularly important as community social work begins to draw domicillary, day care and fieldwork services together in joint community-based programmes – an area of work that surely demands urgent development.

A key question in defining management capability is this: how do the structures, procedures and values of the agency have to change to make them supportive of locally-based forms of work in which the involvement of local people is a central feature? A National Institute publication has indicated the nature of some of these changes: open organisational structures; collective forms of working and supervision; explicit decision-making; the autonomy of local teams; a system of workload, rather than caseload, management; and a role for senior managers as arbitrators and consultants. (For a further discussion of these, see Henderson and Scott, 1984.)

A Last Word

Neighbourhood work, and the efforts of other professionals such as social workers to work in neighbourhoods and to use their resources, are part of the process of developing neighbourhoods as viable social systems. This kind of integrated locality development requires various kinds of interventions and resources; it implies the emergence of a range of networks, linkages and groups – and groups that have a variety of interests from providing services or care, organising leisure or employment facilities to action campaigns about issues that affect people's livelihood.

The antithesis of integrated locality development is both a geographical area composed largely of isolated household units, *and* attempts by professionals to work in a neighbourhood on a single issue, or with a single type of group. Integrated development implies a patchwork of groups and networks (with degrees of overlap in goals and membership) which people can choose, if they so wish, to join for particular puposes at different stages or events in their life. Integrated development does not mean asking residents to declare a 'wholesale' membership to some community identity or ideal; it rather implies the creation of numerous opportunities for people to join with others on a strictly 'limited liability' basis in order to do things of values to themselves and service to others.

At a very basic level, locality development is about putting people in touch with one another, and of promoting their membership in groups and networks. It seeks to develop people's sense of power and significance in acts of association with others that may also achieve an improvement in their social and material well-being. Neighbourhood work is concerned with both political and personal development. At its best, it combines systemic change and individual change. At its most potent, it is concerned not simply with the system or individual, but also with role: it is an intervention that helps people to develop and expand the roles which they have been accustomed to taking, or not taking, in life.

In the act of bringing people together, neighbourhood workers are performing an essential role. They have the much-needed skill of helping people associate with one another in a society where most of the forces at work are to separate and atomise them. As workers put people in touch with one another, it gives priority to those in greatest need, and it is able to do this without stigmatising them.

As long ago as the 1920s, Mary Follet drew out attention to the neighbourhood as 'the inner workshop of democracy'. We are finding today that the neighbourhood can also be the inner workshop of economic regeneration and self-help. We may also take note that not all aspects of our material well-being can be advanced by individual striving and mobility. People need to combine with others to take action on many issues that affect their livelihood, and the necessity for combining together is as evident in neighbourhood as in work-place issues. The many conflicts that are evident on the streets of our inner cities, new towns and peripheral estates indicate the continuing need for a policy of neighbourhood development, and for recognition of the resources and specialist help that may be needed by local people to come together to be more effective in problem solving.

Being a successful worker in a neighbourhood requires a mix of skills, commitment, personal qualities, good luck and much support from one's agency and colleagues. We hope this book gives an indication of the tasks and skills that may be necessary, and that staff and students will find it helpful to make their work more effective, and thus more useful to the local people with whom they are working.

We trust, too, that readers will treat the book as an invitation to contribute, through discussion, research and publication, to a better understanding of neighbourhood work. It is a testing, stressful and complex occupation, particularly in urban areas, and we cannot afford ever to be complacent about the skills and knowledge we offer to agencies and local people.

The recording and writing of neighbourhood workers all too frequently remains within a relatively restricted circulation. The number of mimeographed papers and reports written by workers in order to clarify and communicate what they are doing must be considerable. Yet the fruits of such labour, in terms, for example, of tips, hints, warnings to others – around a range of skill areas – remain buried. Clearly, much of the content of such writing relates only to particular localities and situations, but there will undoubtedly be parts which connect to central themes, problems and achievements of neighbourhood work.

The work of extracting these, and drawing scattered material together, remains a relatively underdeveloped area of neighbourhood work. It is one which we believe deserves more robust treatment. The products might result in neighbourhood workers who are isolated having additional points of guidance and support. Similarly, both community activists and professionals working in the community could turn to less discreet and, at the same time, more tangible guidelines than they have been offered in the past.

We have learned a good deal from accounts of community work provided by practitioners and teachers in this country, the United States and Europe. We have made extensive use of United States and United Kingdom literature in identifying skill components of neighbourhood work. We have also included as many quotations from writing by community workers as space allows.

We have not wanted to produce an academic text, yet nor have we sought to prepare a handbook. There are elements of both in the book, and we hope that it does not fall between two stools as a result. Our intention is that its content be of practical use to neighbourhood workers and others interested in the field. This reflects our interest in recognising and assisting those who are committed to working at the neighbourhood level.

CHAPTER 1

Some Ideas Around Which the Book is Organised

Working in neighbourhoods is still at a point where practitioners, students and activists require guidance, support and clarity in their work. They may want, above all, to extend their understanding of neighbourhood work as a deliberate form of social intervention in communities.

In the same way, agencies which provide services seem anxious to acquire a better grasp of how neighbourhood work is done; and professionals working in the community – doctors, social workers, teachers – seek guidance about an activity or craft which still somewhat eludes their comprehension.

Yet there are more reasons for examining in detail the skills required for practising neighbourhood work. It is possible that unless more work is done and made accessible, the validity of neighbourhood work as a method of intervention will be subject to questioning. If the actions, problems and achievements of workers are not made clear and explicit, then the practice of neighbourhood work will lack rigour. There will be nothing against which to test practice; intuition and charisma will become even more dominant as the touch-stones of good practice than they are already. Society will lose interest in a form of intervention which is inadequately described, analysed and evaluated.

There have been many warnings of the difficulties of integrating theory and practice, and of the dangers of putting too high a value on theory. Yet there remains wide scope to produce more material about neighbourhood work with the right kind of 'mix' between theory and practice, thereby yielding frameworks which are both valid and relevant.

In bringing out the first edition in 1980, our aim was to make a modest contribution primarily from a practice base. Our hunch

18

was that this approach, with its emphasis on a detailed exposition of a range of skills in clearly defined neighbourhood situations, was exploring relatively unchartered territory.

One inspiration for the first edition was the work done with practitioners on five day-release workshops. These were held between 1976 and 1979 with the purpose of identifying and then improving skills used in neighbourhood work. The workshops produced valuable material upon which we have not hesitated to draw in writing this book.

The Lonely Cyclist

One problem often faced by workers is the isolated nature of their jobs. There are rarely opportunities for a team approach. Sometimes they work as a 'specialist' member of a team of social workers or other professionals, but they often lack the close support of colleagues working on the same task. If they want that kind of support they usually have to make a point of deliberately acquiring it from co-workers who have different tasks; winning their interest and trust can take time. Even so, most workers are in an agency or project of some kind, and one implication of this is that most worker's jobs will be within a prior policy context not created by themselves. Part of the work of 'situating oneself' which we look at in the next chapter involves understanding, adjusting to and influencing this policy context.

However, professional isolation also takes hold of many neighbourhood workers by the very nature of the work they do. They appear to have roving agendas for each day, moving swiftly between contrasting scenarios: a meeting with the chairman of the adventure playground association; booking a van for a jumble sale; time in the local library to collect information; helping a group carry out a survey; an interview with a planning officer about a possible housing improvement area. The worker often has to handle such situations within a short space of time, and he or she is therefore always working with different audiences and constituencies from varied role positions.

This is a theme we shall return to; it makes an interesting contrast, for instance, to the 'public' nature of the worker's job done at meetings, demonstrations and social events. Here we draw attention to the 'loner' position into which the worker is forced, constantly moving between systems, and the effect this has of rationing time for reflection, recording and writing about work; these too are tasks which normally require solitude, and the priority need is very often to find support from other neighbourhood workers.

The Neighbourhood

We have already discussed the significance of neighbourhood in the introduction, and we now want to make a few additional comments here. It has now become conventional wisdom among neighbourhood workers to acknowledge the limited impact their work at a local level can have on basic problems such as inadequate housing, unemployment and poverty. These are the result of structural causes at regional, national and international levels, and they will be changed, it is argued, only through overt political action at wider levels than the neighbourhood.

This line of thought is often linked to arguments that community workers and community groups should work through the Labour movement in order to bring about social change. Sometimes the effect is to persuade neighbourhood workers away from the small-scale, detailed work with groups in order to put their energies into influencing social and economic policies through existing political channels.

At the same time, those who wish to continue neighbourhood work are often forced, because of these structuralist arguments, to think through their position more rigorously. This challenge is very healthy. It makes it necessary, for example, that workers be precise about the significance of the neighbourhood, why it is important and to whom, and about what neighbourhood consists of. It also obliges them to be honest and realistic about the extent of social change that can be achieved through neighbourhood work.

Finally, criticism of the insignificance of neighbourhood work as a tool for major social change require those who remain committed to working in the neighbourhood to be positive and open about their values and objectives: they need to make explicit their belief that helping a community to live and grow, combating the tendency of residents to turn in on themselves at the risk of fragmenting their communities, are tasks of major significance which must continue to be done. The often limited nature of these tasks within the overall social system does not result in their being any less important. The arguments for working at neighbourhood level are manifold, but they need to be articulated and supported with evidence. An analogous comment has been made by Chris Holmes in relation to housing:

> Those who argue for a radically different approach to inner city problems . . . are right to stress the structural causes, income inequalities and diminishing employment opportunities which have caused the rundown of inner city areas. Area-based housing programmes alone cannot reverse these forces. But we must be wary of dismissing them as irrelevant. Too many areas suffered through the 1950s and 1960s from comprehensive, centrally administered redevelopment strategies. No inner city policies will work unless they are rooted in the experience and aspirations of small neighbourhoods, shaped and controlled by their representatives and administered by officials working within the area they serve. (1977)

Neighbourhood workers attach similar importance to the interaction of individuals, families and groups within local communities. There is a need to nurture the right of community groups to express themselves and to participate in decision- and policy-making.

The term neighbourhood work has been adopted for three reasons. First, it gives the subject of our writing a clear categorisation within the practice of community work. We use 'neighbourhood work' to refer to direct face-to-face work with local people who have formed groups or networks to tackle a need or problem they have identified, to give support to each other and/or to provide services to people in the area. This definition separates neighbourhood work from the two other strands of community work: social planning and agency change and development. Occasionally we make use of the term community work; for the purposes of this book it is interchangeable with neighbourhood work.

The second reason for favouring the term neighbourhood work has to do with what it implies. We do not wish to give neighbourhood work a wholly geographical definition. For one thing neighbourhood cannot be stated exactly; a worker may be active in a number of neighbourhoods which are coterminous. More important, we do not wish to argue that because a worker is engaged primarily at neighbourhood level he or she cannot or should not be actively involved with wider concerns, whether these be city-wide or national.

Yet we are anxious to capture that connotation of neighbourhood which means close, face-to-face work with people committed to their community. The substance of interventions by neighbourhood workers entails working intimately with territorial groups; work with groups which share a common interest across a wider area occupies less of workers' time, although we do not underestimate the significance of this work (see Chapter 9).

Ideas developed about neighbourhood forums of one kind or another are relevant to a discussion of neighbourhood work. According to a Department of the Environment booklet on neighbourhood councils, 'experience suggests that a council should ideally consist of between 6,000 and 10,000 people, though there are no rigid limits' (1977), while the original brief for the CDPs recommended project localities of 10,000 to 20,000 population. In emphasising the geographical focus of neighbourhood work we are aware that we may court the wrath of sociologists of communities, even though we do not imply that a neighbourhood worker or community group should feel 'imprisoned' by geographical boundaries, or that problems or issues facing small neighbourhoods necessarily originate within them.

The practice of neighbourhood work assumes that the neighbourhood has some importance for people. It will mean more to some than to others. There will, for example, be significant cultural and regional differences. The point is often made too that a large amount of neighbourhood work is undertaken with women; because they frequently have no choice, neighbourhood action speaks directly to their situation.

Encouraging local people to work collectively is an aspect of the struggle to give real meaning to the concept of democracy. Neighbourhood work seeks to involve people at grass-roots level in decisions and policies which affect them and their neighbourhoods. There is the expectation, too, that activity in neighbourhoods around a range of social, economic and political issues will permeate and influence other decision-making arenas.

Finally, the term neighbourhood work suggests to us a job for which a range of explicit, hard skills are required in order to work effectively and sensitively with local people. We are not interested in 'professionalising' community work, but we do believe that local people want the service and support of skilled community workers, just as they want skilled doctors, skilled caretakers and skilled plumbers. Doing community work more professionally in this sense should not be confused with debates about the professionalisation of a group of workers.

Seeing Neighbourhood Work as a Process

We have found it valuable to see neighbourhood work as a process. The usefulness of a process account is to make explicit the variety of tasks that workers carry out in their work with neighbourhood groups. The act of establishing process provides a way of *identifying, distinguishing, ordering* and *categorising* the activities of the neighbourhood worker. *Identifying* the elements of practice is of help in alerting the worker to what needs to be done in his or her work. In particular, the worker may see the varying needs of groups at different stages of the process, and this in turn may be suggestive of the different roles, skills and knowledge likely to be required of the worker. Additionally, *distinguishing* the different aspects of neighbourhood work may help those responsible for training, support and supervision better to identify the ways in which they can contribute to the skill development of students and practitioners.

The *ordering* of the elements of practice turns our attention to the timing, sequencing and interrelatedness of the worker's interventions. Specifically, the act of ordering the parts of work reveals the necessity for planning the worker's activities. For example, success in carrying out the end-phase of neighbourhood work is contingent upon decisions the worker makes, or fails to make, at the beginning of the intervention. Attempts at evaluation may be frustrated because of inattention in the early phases to setting up appropriate recording procedures; the kind of withdrawal a worker makes from a group may be determined by the kind of role established *vis-à-vis* the group since the first contact with them.

The *categorising* of neighbourhood work practice not only imposes 'order' on the various activities that comprise the worker's day-to-day practice but also facilitates the identification of similarities in the work of different practitioners engaged with groups from different neighbourhoods pursuing a range of issues. The ability to categorise our work, and to generalise from it, is an important step towards the development of a practice theory in neighbourhood work.

A process view of neighbourhood work also leads us to the dynamic of our interventions. Through process accounts we may better understand the *purposeful* nature of our work. The fact that the interventions of workers have intentionality and direction is important to grasp because in the actual doing of neighbourhood work practitioners often feel caught in a turbulent environment of community activities with little immediate sense of where their work is leading them, or the group with whom they work.

Of course, the working situation for the neighbourhood worker very often *is* unpredictable and confusing. The ability to conceive of one's activity at any point in time as part of an on-going process provides not only sense and direction but the opportunities to disengage and stand back from the action. We suggest that the activity of 'taking stock' is an important element in the process of neighbourhood work.

The View of a Stranger

Let us suppose that a Person from Mars visits one of our cities, and finds herself on the pavement of a busy street. She becomes curious about the meaning of an activity that we know as driving. She guesses there is some individual or even collective purpose behind this activity; she stops passers-by in order to discover the meaning of it. If her appearance and manner do not inhibit conversation, she may be told that driving is a way of getting people and goods from A to B; and that most of the drivers will have some purpose related to business or pleasure. She may be given more abstract explanations of driving that, for example, define its place in economic processes of production, distribution and consumption; or in social processes such as maintaining the links between nuclear and extended parts of a family. Some pedestrians might raise several issues about driving – for example, about pollution, energy expenditure and safety.

24

Our visitor may become dissatisfied with these kinds of explanation. 'These people have told me *about* driving', she reflects, 'but no one has told me *how to do it*.' This would be a fair comment if she herself wanted to drive with competence and be able to teach others how to drive. 'These "know-about" statements', she muses, 'are extremely interesting and important; but my priority is to learn to drive. I therefore need someone who can talk to me in terms of "know-how" propositions.'

The Person from Mars then seeks people who can explain driving in terms of a series of tasks, such as opening the car door; getting in; adjusting seat and mirror; fastening seat belts; locating and switching-on ignition; selection of gear; release of hand-brake; and so on, until tasks are outlined for driving, stopping and parking the car. Explanations of this kind would be best suited to teaching the Person from Mars how to drive; although explanations using 'know-about' propositions might also be needed. For example, it might help her to appreciate better the tasks of locking and unlocking doors, to understand these tasks in relation to societal issues like deviancy and the unequal distribution of wealth and access to consumer goods. We might even give her Huw Beynon's 1975 book *Working for Ford*, though she may find exploring the issues it raises so compelling that she gives herself insufficient time to master the practice of driving.

For most people, the primary interest is knowing *how* to drive rather than knowing *about* driving. In neighbourhood work, however, there is as powerful an interest in 'know-about' propositions and discussions. Community work is directly and energetically concerned with the causes, but more often with the manifestations, of major social and economic problems in society; it is then only proper that its practitioners, students and teachers, want to discuss matters *about* community work, and particularly questions about its goals and functions, the nature of its place in society and its contribution to the amelioration of poverty, powerlessness and lack of opportunity among some of society's members, groups and classes.

In the last chapter of the book, we develop further the differences between 'know-how', 'know-why' and 'know-about' propositions. At this stage, however, we want only to indicate that the idea of process is a useful way to deal with 'know-how' material in neighbourhood work.

25

We present below our account of the process of neighbourhood work that provides the structure for the remainder of this book. Our treatment of some of the initial stages of this process reflects its urban origin, and readers interested, for example, in rural, suburban or new town environments must adapt and add to our discussion in order to increase its relevance to these situations. We believe that our discussion of ideas and principles pertains to a variety of work environments, even though the *examples* which we use to illustrate our points may be too predominantly urban for the satisfaction of some readers.

Our nine-stage process of neighbourhood work is as follows:

(1) entering the neighbourhood;
(2) getting to know the neighbourhood;
(3) what next? needs, goals and roles;
(4) making contacts and bringing people together;
(5) forming and building organisations;
(6) helping to clarify goals and priorities;
(7) keeping the organisation going;
(8) dealing with friends and enemies;
(9) leavings and endings.

A few points about this process: it does not portray the phases through which a group, or a neighbourhood, moves, though there is some discussion of group development and process in Chapter 8. Our process rather identifies the major tasks, or areas of work, in which the worker is involved. This is not to say that each piece of neighbourhood work will necessarily and always involve the worker in these major tasks; we believe that every worker in each piece of neighbourhood work will be involved in some of these phases and tasks, and that our process defines the major areas of work that any worker will be engaged in if he or she sees some neighbourhood action through from beginning to end.

There are clearly a good many interconnections between each of the stages in this process. In practice, the stages do not represent discrete categories of tasks, skills and knowledge. The activities of each stage prepare for, and feed into, the subsequent stages; and there is, and ought to be, feedback from each stage to the worker about what he or she (and others) have achieved in preceding stages. Some of the stages continue as on-going tasks for the community worker: for example, the activities of data collection and making contacts are ever-present responsibilities for the worker, and are usually improved both qualitatively and quantitively by a worker's tasks in stages of the process that are, in our account, subsequent to them. In brief, the process is not a simple sequential or linear one; most of the stages occur simultaneously with one or some of the others.

We believe that our account of the process of neighbourhood work provides a basic kit of words, ideas and frameworks. As with most kits, it is our hope that readers will play around with it, adding and subtracting bits, in order to produce something that is more suited to their needs and interests. A kit, after all, is only as good as the shapes and functions to which its users can put it.

The process will certainly have to be adapted by those working in neighbourhoods who wish to set up networks, neighbourhood care schemes or programmes involving the use of volunteers. Guidelines for setting up, maintaining and evaluating neighbourhood care schemes have been produced by ADVANCE, a London-based agency providing advice and training in this area (see Hedley *et al.*, 1985).

There is the danger that too much will be expected of the neighbourhood work process. The reader will have noted that – for reasons of space – we have neglected, or only given slight attention to, some key skill areas for neighbourhood work: recording, supervision and evaluation come into this category. It is essential both that workers obtain such knowledge and skill and remain aware of the need to update it. Neighbourhood work, like mountain streams which ceaselessly seek out new nooks and crannies, has to provoke energy, interest and a sense of excitement. Much of neighbourhood work's strength comes from its search for more effective and meaningful methods, tactics and strategies. Without this, it risks becoming arid and moribund.

The neighbourhood work process should be seen as a tool. It is not the only available analytical framework and, as is the habit with some tools, we are conscious that in time its usefulness may diminish. In addition it should be stressed that by itself the process account is quite insufficient for doing neighbourhood work. Values, ideology and creativity constitute the lifeblood of organising and action at local level. They require that anger, caring, determination and a host of other emotions and expressions of commitment be part of the daily vocabulary of neighbourhood workers. The process model has to lie alongside these, not dominate them.

It is possible to combine writing practice theory for neighbourhood work with an explicit value framework. Kahn (1970), for example, writes about neighbourhood work in this way. We chose to offer something closer to a 'textbook' approach chiefly because of a concern that the material should be applied as widely as possible. We suggest that there are identifiable skills and techniques which can be used in a multiplicity of situations regardless of the value stance of workers or neighbourhood groups. At the same time we insist upon the centrality of values for any neighbourhood intervention.

A Work Book

There is a need for anyone involved in neighbourhood work – local people, full-time workers, trainers – to be more forward-looking about it. Merely responding to changes of circumstance or demands becomes weakening and does not help the practice of neighbourhood work to improve. This is one reason why we conceived of this book as a work book. We have tried to make the material easily accessible; each of the following chapters starts with a summary of its major areas of content.

We have also worked on the assumption that readers will want to change the book, amending and adding to it according to their experience and their ideas about how practice should develop.

It may be, for example, that people will want to expand those parts which deal with the day-to-day work with community groups and their management; at present the balance of the material is weighted more towards planning an intervention, making contact and forming groups. We would encourage people to wrestle with the book in that way and would be pleased to hear from them about their experience of using the book and about their ideas for changing it.

Neighbourhood workers are often tempted to tackle every situation which they encounter, and many times they are under pressure to do so. Training seeks to counter this tendency. One of its main purposes is constantly to confront students with the question 'why?'. Why are you planning to carry out a survey? Why are you attending every meeting of such-and-such a group? The legitimacy of making such challenges lies in the belief that standing back from the action, examining a piece of work critically with the help of someone who is to an extent outside it, will result in more thoughtful and therefore more effective work being accomplished. It is a similar line of thinking which informs our ideas of how this book might be used in training.

Is it all a bit too much?

We take the reader through most of the main phases of the process. A worker will often draw upon the same knowledge and skills for different parts of the process, and we try to indicate this. The occasional reappearance of material in chapters, or reference to skills already identified, is therefore not repetitive.

We often wondered when writing this book whether it might appear too detailed and comprehensive. There is a danger that we elaborate the process of neighbourhood work so much as to discourage anyone from embarking on it. Perhaps we have provided prescriptions which no one will feel he or she has the skills, energy and time to follow in practice.

We must stress, therefore, that what we have written should be used more as a source of ideas on particular points rather than read through at one sitting. For example, trainers and students may read a chapter as a preparation for discussing and extending specific skills through role play and video; this might be followed by a seminar on the issues that have emerged from the chapter and the workshop; and this discussion might in turn be followed by further reading.

We have referred already to the workshops on neighbourhood work skills. We anticipate this book can be used in training courses of that kind; these in turn need to dovetail with other educational methods. We shall briefly describe the nature of the workshops because they illustrate the importance of enabling students to partialise their learning about neighbourhood work as opposed to tackling it all at once; we also wish to emphasise the desirability of combining experiential learning about neighbourhood work with more 'intellectual' forms of learning.

The workshops are organised around a number of role-play

exercises, decided upon by the participants. The situations in neighbourhood work that are invariably chosen are micro-episodes such as making contact with residents by door-knocking or in a pub; going with a deputation of residents to, say, a funder or a local authority committee; handling incidents in community groups such as the disruptive or over-talkative or domineering member, or events such as the expression of racism.

The workshop participants work themselves on developing the scenario for the role play, allocating roles and getting people into role through discussion and rehearsal. The role play is then enacted, usually lasting for about five minutes; there is usually too much in anything that goes over ten minutes.

The role play is videotaped and then replayed to the participants. A discussion follows that focuses on the way in which the worker in the role play carried out his tasks and role; the object is to highlight those things the worker did well and badly, that affected his relationship with 'community residents' and his success in achieving the goals the worker had set himself. The role play is then acted and videotaped again (perhaps two or three times) so that enhanced performance develops as a result of discussion and of self-learning that occurs as people see themselves on television. Video is a powerful medium for learning, and the work of the trainer is to ensure that it, and subsequent discussion, are used creatively to improve competence and understanding in some of the situations in which neighbourhood workers find themselves. The advantages of using video in role play for skills training in social work education are discussed by McCaughan and Scott (1978). Their observation that the trainer does not need to dominate the feedback discussion to make educational points, because the material is available for all to work at, is especially relevant to neighbourhood work skills training.

Reading about skills can be interspersed with doing role play with video. In that way, students can handle better the quantity of knowledge they meet, and examine it critically. This is only one illustration of integrating the book with other educational methods. We would be most interested to hear from trainers and students of their experiences of using the book, out of curiosity but also from a concern to help generate valid practice theories for doing neighbourhood work. For that to happen, critical appraisal and sharing are essential.

CHAPTER 2

Entering the Neighbourhood

Thinking About Going In
    Orientation
    Values and roles
    Planning and problem analysis

Negotiating Entry
    Existing community groups
    Agencies
    The worker's agency

How a worker starts the succession of steps which gains him access to a neighbourhood is of critical importance. The 'way in' as suggested by Cowan has to be thought through rigorously:

> In a three or four year community development programme, the starting point is like the opening moves in a game of chess: it determines what kind of game will be played. It is a distinct and crucial stage in a piece of 'change-work'. (1979)

This chapter examines the kind of preliminary thinking and action which needs to take place. We call these *thinking about going in*, and *negotiating entry*. All of it is still very much in the pre-action phase of neighbourhood work. The question of whether or not a worker will 'go in' at all to a neighbourhood remains legitimate and relevant throughout.

Thinking About Going In

The motivation to throw yourself quickly into some form of practical activity is normally strong. This is true both of workers newly appointed to posts and of established workers starting projects in a neighbourhood where they have not worked before. The expression and satisfaction of the 'doing' of neighbourhood work, compared to thinking and talking about it, entices even the most experienced workers to move rapidly into seeking out and working with people.

31

4223

In many respects this tendency is as unsurprising as it is welcome: workers who are not eager about finding out how people express community needs, or who do not genuinely enjoy working closely with a multiplicity and variety of local people, are unlikely to stay with neighbourhood work for long. The themes of felt and expressed needs and of working alongside people rather than simply on their behalf lie at the heart of a worker's involvement in the neighbourhood.

The stage before contact begins consists of a combination of orientation by the worker to her surroundings and of building-up a plan of entry into the neighbourhood. It involves avoiding making decisions too early on, while at the same time maintaining antennae which are constantly alert to useful information, leads, contacts and potential allies.

The questions which the worker needs to have at the front of her mind at this stage are: what kind of work should I do? what are the best ways of helping me do it? how should I set about getting there? The formulation of such questions is an essential antecedent for neighbourhood workers. An important influence on their formulation should be a worker's thinking about what he or she learnt from the last job, project or campaign, although this should be done critically – workers can get 'stuck' with an early success and keep trying to repeat it. We distinguish the following as being central to a worker's consideration: *orientation*, *values and roles* and *planning and problem analysis*.

Orientation

Neighbourhood workers inevitably have to know and work with a range of professionals, in varied organisational settings. The nature of their work forces them into this position. They will usually need to know, and be known by, a range of organisations and individuals in the areas where they work. They tend to become walking encyclopaedias of relevant, up-to-date information about who's who and where to go in the neighbourhoods and in the organisations which serve them.

Anyone who intends to become seriously involved in a neighbourhood must set time aside for absorbing the nature of the neighbourhood and the attitudes and interests of both local people and professional colleagues. The worker can always correct and improve initial impressions later. The importance of this initial scanning lies in awakening the worker's senses to the number and range of factors to be considered before moving into action. Orientation thus becomes an essential preliminary to planning intervention in the neighbourhood.

As far as the community aspect is concerned, it can mean simply walking about an area – a stranger literally taking the first steps towards eventual partnership with local people. It is best if workers vary the times of the day and night at which they make such forays, for then they will be more likely to absorb an accurate, albeit sketchy, picture. When workers engage in such walking about they must be careful not to confuse it with more detailed and deliberate observation and contact-making in the community, both of which are distinct phases which come later. The worker's incursions into the community at this stage are to assist in deciding how to plan an intervention; they come strictly in the pre-planning phase.

Characteristics of the neighbourhood to be noticed are: degrees of traffic densities in different streets, condition and types of housing, the extent of untidiness and vandalism, the existence of open space, the location of factories, offices, pubs and shops, and the availability of public transport. The worker might note too some obvious features about people in the area: old people walking uphill with their shopping, the presence of a racially mixed population, or simply the ebb and flow of people at different times of day.

Some of the impressions will merely reaffirm what the worker has been told already by colleagues, while others will be new; it will depend a lot on whether the worker is starting a new piece of work in the area, or whether he is joining an existing programme for which there are background papers and reports. Whether the messages a worker receives are old or new when he familiarises himself with the area and with the life-styles of its residents, they form a key part of his orientation.

The effort of tuning into the organisational context of the job demands, first of all, that workers begin to obtain a grasp of agency functioning. They will usually start with their own agency and then broaden out to acquire an initial understanding of organisations which either operate alongside their own agency or which they know are likely to impinge in some way on the neighbourhood where they intend to work. There are a number of further actions that workers need to take in relation to organisations and we discuss these later in the chapter.

A final component of the orientation phase incorporates both the community and the agency; this is an awareness of the social, economic and political climate in which the practitioner is to do neighbourhood work. It is most easily illustrated by taking extreme examples. Bryant, for instance, in a talk to community work teachers at York in 1976, explained why community work in Glasgow almost inevitably is taken up with conflicts over housing owing to the severity of housing problems there. Any worker new to that city will pick this up quickly and thereby anticipate the mood and focus of community groups and the likely relationships with the housing authorities. In the same way, community workers in Belfast clearly face exceptional problems of latent and overt communal violence and a unique political situation. A contrasting example of a context implicitly imposing a framework is the position of a worker in a traditional rural community which may be resistant to any outside attempts made to introduce changes.

It is possible for a worker to identify sets of attitudes which permeate the area where he or she is due to work, and the organisations to be met. The urban/rural contrast will be one determinant, as will the overall extent of relative affluence or deprivation. As each day passes, the worker will be adding to his store of knowledge on these and other points, tightening up initial perceptions or assumptons. At some point the worker is likely to want to set time aside for methodical study of some of these by, for example, examination of an area's social history. In the initial stages of his work, however, it is as if he must lay himself open to receiving the hidden messages and assumptions in the commuity and its institutions, exploring political, social and economic complexities. This is likely to help workers to pitch the character and form of their interventions in a neighbourhood at the right level. It will be particularly relevant for when they first approach existing community groups. What the worker sees, and the interpretations he makes, will inevitably be subjective at this stage. Equally, first impressions will not always be entirely accurate.

Values and Roles

In planning intervention in a neighbourhood the worker needs to spend time clarifying his or her own position on key value issues. Before they have substantial contact with a community they need to have clarified their thinking on major questions of value and ideology. The decisions they take once they move into a neighbourhood will be partly determined by their values and by their perception of role. They must have a stance on both of these, and be ready to articulate them when necessary. The authors of *Principles and Practice of Community Work in a British Town* remind us that the worker does not appear in a community out of a vacuum:

> On the contrary, he arrives there with both pre-conceptions and, as a rule, past experience of similar work. Though he will try to approach the problems of a community in a neutral spirit, letting the particular problems and demands of the situation present themselves as far as possible, nevertheless he cannot help but have a set of conceptual expectations, theoretical and practical, which affect his actions. (Taylor *et al.*, 1976)

We shall do no more here than list five questions which relate to values and role. Our prime interest is to identify some of the relevant questions to be aware of *before* the worker starts to make contact with the community. There are several others, and they are bound to vary in significance for each person. We present a fuller discussion of some of these matters in Chapter 4.

Process/Product A continuing dilemma is whether your interest lies essentially in assisting the self-learning process of individuals through their participation in community groups, or whether it focuses on the achievement of specific tasks which can bring material or psychological benefits to neighbourhoods. If workers favour a combination fo the two, how do they attempt to maintain a balance, and how do they handle the difficulties which arise when process and product goals come into conflict – as they will do? The worker has to see the intricate connection between the two. Closely linked to this question is that of time-scale, of how long or short a time commitment a worker will make to a neighbourhood.

Consideration of these questions implies, in effect, that a worker will have conceptualised a philosophy and set of objectives for working at the neighbourhood level. It should include analysis of the links that neighbourhood work can make between local and national issues, between his or her involvement in practice at neighbourhood level and the wider social and economic policies which affect the locality.

Rationalism/Intuition   It is tempting to suggest that the most effective workers are those who act and behave as themselves in neighbourhood work; they have a natural instinct to follow the right paths. There is no distinction between themselves as persons and themselves as neighbourhood workers. Those who lack this intuitive quality, it might be argued, are obliged to depend on analysis of particular situations before they act.

While this is a caricature of two types of approach to neighbourhood work, there do seem to be workers who have a natural ability to handle issues in an intuitive manner. There are few of them, and even the most skilled of them would be unlikely to decry the usefulness of rigorous analysis. Most neighbourhood workers, however, need to acquire a number of skills, and develop particular qualities in order to be effective in their work. Furthermore, they depend on being able to use analytic tools and a rational process to assist them in their tasks. It is probably helpful for workers to assess where they put themselves on the intuitive and rationalist continuum before they start functioning in a neighbourhood.

The style in which they operate will affect the kind of projects workers choose to develop, as well as the support mechanisms they will require. They need to have an idea of their own strengths and weaknesses as individuals if they are to perform effectively; all workers make abundant use of themselves as people and of the human qualities they possess. Furthermore workers may have to develop human qualities for the benefit of their work which they may never have used.

Participation   It is recognised that theories of participation are of direct relevance to neighbourhood workers, with the proviso that a high degree of participation is not always appropriate or sufficient for bringing about major changes in a community. A worker may often be forced to choose between the effectiveness of a small group of people working on a task, set against an awareness of the importance of expanding such a group's membership. He has to be aware of this potential disjunction of aims, which he is likely to face frequently. One criterion which can be used is the degree to which a group's membership is added to and renewed. Groups with small membership may still represent a constituency, but groups which consist of self-perpetuating cliques have moved a long way from the participatory goals of community work.

Leadership Neighbourhood workers are rapidly put in the position of having to accept, parry or reject requests to them from individuals and groups in the community to take on leadership roles. While neighbourhood work aims to enable local people to assume leadership in a multiplicity of situations, it may be appropriate to the methods and strategies of a neighbourhood worker for him to play a leadership role as an interim measure. We shall suggest that this is particularly likely in situations where the formation of a group is difficult and time-consuming, and where a worker can legitimately demonstrate leadership skills or give confidence to a group by providing it with direction.

Since workers can safely anticipate being put under pressure to provide leadership, it is necessary for them to crystallise their response beforehand. The same applies to the style of work they intend to adopt and the role they favour (we examine these in detail in Chapter 4). When they change role it is important to convey a clear impression of who they are and what they are doing. This area is particularly important when the variability of the membership of community groups is considered. For example, experience suggests how easy it is for male workers to fall into a stereotyped relationship with women in a group. Remfrey (1979) refers to the bantering and joking which can take place but which can conceal an essentially sexist divide between a male worker and female group members. Gallagher (1977) has written helpfully on this question. Our point here is to alert workers to the issue before work with groups begins. Similar advice applies to white workers: they need to think about how they relate to black members of groups (see Thomas, 1986).

Accountability In the event of a conflict of interest arising between a worker's agency and a group he supports, the worker needs to have ready a set of arguments to underpin whatever position is taken. Even when no conflict arises, a worker experiences tension between his agency and the community's interests, although this will vary according to the kind of agency in which he is employed. For example, a neighbourhood worker is always aware of the danger of giving away too much information to those in power about community groups and their ways of working.

The question of accountability of workers relates closely to the ethics of intervention in a community. Both are issues which workers have to think about carefully. It is certain that the rigour and clarity of the thinking will be put to the test in the work situation; it is exceptional for neighbourhood workers to remain onlookers.

It is worth noting again that most workers will find themselves as members of an agency, a project or a community work team. Thus the worker will not have a blank cheque but will be held to account for his work by fellow team members and agency management.

In itemising the above issues surrounding the subjects of values and role, we emphasise again that we have sought only to identify key ideas and not to develop them. Their study and debate must form an essential part of any work in a neighbourhood, and our decision merely to list them should not be taken as undervaluing either their significance or their complexity.

Planning and Problem Analysis

It will be seen that the emphasis we give to planning entry into a neighbourhood is upon the value of reflection and orientation especially in relation to a worker's values and role. It has to do with the nature of the work which is going to be undertaken, and the attitudes the worker takes with him or her when starting to know a neighbourhood. It is the stage in the neighbourhood work process when workers will have most time to think at this level without interruption and without being overinfluenced by their involvement. Once they are working on projects and issues in the neighbourhood, the pressures of time and competing needs, demands and events will prejudice their ability to do such reflective thinking.

The development of a plan of entry must include what Ross (1967) calls 'the process of locating and defining a problem (or set of problems)'. It is important to stress the spiral-like movement of problem analysis and action, each being informed by the other as work proceeds. The bursts of activity in neighbourhood work and the rapid accumulation of tasks, meetings and contacts can conceal attempts made deliberately to follow steps in a process even if the steps cannot be sequential.

We agree, however, with Perlman and Gurin (1972) that 'Organising people to achieve social change requires planning to guide both the ends and means of their efforts'. A major component in the worker's pre-planning phase is the identification of the categories of activities and tasks which have to be undertaken and which will enable the worker to begin building up a description of a neighbourhood's problems. He will then be in a position to analyse the problems, and from there formulate a plan of action.

Too close an equation of developing a plan of intervention with problem analysis of a neighbourhood carries with it a danger of implying entirely negative characteristics of the local environment and of the people who live there. Any such tendency should certainly be avoided. Neighbourhood workers try, above all, to seek out and nourish the strengths and resources of local communities and shun any suggestions of labelling.

Our argument up to this point is that neighbourhood workers, having spent time on reflection and orientation, have to begin to sharpen their ideas about what they intend to do. This can be achieved by them finding out and broadly categorising the problems facing a neighbourhood, and thence devising a plan of intervention. Closely linked to this work is the need for workers to obtain initial legitimacy for their plans and future presence.

Negotiating Entry

In the past, community workers sometimes used the device of involving themselves with short-term or relatively minor activities in a neighbourhood with the purpose of using them to open up contacts for working on more major issues and problems – it does not, of course, always work. This approach might be called the direct way into working with the community. While it can have distinct tactical advantages, we consider that, if it is not preceded or accompanied by more searching and explicit moves by the worker to begin the neighbourhood work process, it is likely to be counter-productive.

We call this work negotiating entry, and suggest that it can be differentiated from later steps of gathering data and building up contacts. Clearly, in negotiating entry, the worker does collect data and meet people. The chief difference is that, while the last two are related directly to engagement in a neighbourhood, negotiating entry is concerned with clearing a pathway which will facilitate that engagement.

An example of the direct way in, through immediate contact via activity, is the following extract of a worker's initial period in a Family Service Units project:

> I found that my involvement in the summer project was a most successful way of introducing myself to people in the street and I was probably accepted much more readily by both children and adults than if I had had to make myself known by knocking on doors. However, my involvement in the project meant that I had virtually cut myself off from the Unit and after the end of the summer I spent a large proportion of my time at the Unit so that I could gain support from being a member of the team. (1974)

Clearly, such an approach will be successful in many instances as a means of generating a work programme, and we shall see later (Chapter 5) how informal contact-making constitutes a crucial part of the worker's task once she has formulated a plan of action. We believe, however, that there are dangers in relying on it at an early stage in neighbourhood work. It reduces the possibility of the worker forming a reasonably accurate picture of the area, and the people and organisations in it, *before committing himself or herself to any action*. It can also distract workers from opening up communications with key agencies – including their own – which already have a presence in the area.

Furthermore, it is the experience of many workers that, once committed to a line of action with existing groups, or even with

40

those in the process of formation, it becomes very difficult for them to draw back and start afresh with different groups or a new constituency. Too early an engagement may result in workers finding themselves supporting groups with which, at a later stage, they would prefer not to be so closely involved, or from which they would actually like to dissociate themselves.

In practice, the worker will frequently become involved with an existing community activity as a means of entering the community at the same time that she is drawing up an ordered and selected snapshot of the area as a prelude to formulating a plan. Or the worker will latch on to an obvious need which can begin to be met swiftly.

Negotiating entry demands rigorous thinking on the part of the worker along with some preliminary and minimal contact with community leaders and professional workers. We are conscious of the risk of being over-prescriptive in a field of activity which is characterised by great diversity. There are, in particular, major differences here for a worker depending on whether she is employed by a statutory or voluntary agency. For example, a person employed in a three- or four-person voluntary project will often be committed to a more collective form of policy and decision-making than the worker located in a large statutory organisation and clearly that will shape the kind of thinking and planning undertaken at this stage.

The role involves the following components:

- requesting and selecting information
- presentation of credentials
- self-introduction and introduction of others.

We shall now examine the extent to which workers use these and other skills, and how they do so, in the three major arenas where they will do their work in this phase: *existing community groups*, *relevant agencies* and *their own agency*.

Existing Community Groups

A worker may plan to operate in a neighbourhood where someone has not worked before, or she may be due to enter an area which has already experienced the intervention of one or more

41

neighbourhood workers. Whichever it is, an awareness that boundaries are about to be crossed is essential. This is true in the psychological, political and the geographical sense of boundary. Until a worker begins to gain the trust of individuals, families, existing leadership and groups in a community he or she is as much an intruder there as any stranger would be. Thomas has described how the community worker, even more than the new postman, milkman or caretaker, is a stranger to the tenants of an estate:

> The new postman may have a strange face, but his function is known and accepted by the tenants. The community worker, however, is distinguished both by his class position and by the fact that his function is not understood by the tenants. (1975b)

The writings of Newman (1972) and Jacobs (1972) contain valuable material for neighbourhood workers who are planning a fresh piece of intervention, reminding them in particular to be aware of existing collective identities in neighbourhoods. Attention is drawn to this point in order to underline the sensitivity and listening skills upon which neighbourhood workers have to draw as they start to discover the complex workings of a community and begin to obtain recognition from parts of it. Workers will be as much under observation, and being tested out, as observing and exploring the community themselves.

The process of reaching toward mutual recognition is very much a two-way affair, otherwise it will be impossible for workers to establish an identity with a community. At its most simple level, this means a worker giving local people the opportunity to see her, to put her in a context without feeling any obligation to begin work with her. This is close to the classic community development approach of spending a great deal of time being publicly visible, exemplified by the writing of Batten, and by the work of Ilys Booker in Notting Dale:

> Ilys' conscious tactics were to be seen about the area, to walk on a worked-out basis so that she arrived at the school gates about the time the mothers were taking or fetching the children; to go to the launderette and sit about and talk there; to look at the area as she walked round so that she had a mental picture of the kind of people and what they did; to get her face familiar to

them and theirs to her. She spent a long time doing this and saw it as part of her work. She must have walked several miles a day when she started. (Quoted in Mitton and Morrison, 1972)

The point to note about 'putting oneself about' an area is its deliberate and unhaphazard nature. For this reason, phrases sometimes used loosely by neighbourhood workers such as 'hanging about the area for a few weeks', 'wandering around' or 'getting the feel of the place' should be adopted guardedly. There are specific objectives for the worker in spending time on establishing a presence in a neighbourhood, and of course they extend beyond just the physical presence of the worker. They include, in particular, introduction and first meetings with a range of local people.

There are numerous ways by which neighbourhood workers arrive at the point of intending to work in neighbourhoods, and we do not propose to catalogue them. For example, a worker does not necessarily choose the most deprived of neighbourhoods within a deprived area. He or she might consider a locality which has the most community action potential in order to set an example. Resources for holding meetings, or the neighbourhood's accessibility to the worker's base, or the attitude of existing community groups could all be taken into account in making a choice.

We shall indicate the kind of action a worker is likely to take in three familiar forms of intervention: a worker assigned to work in a particular neighbourhood by his employing agency, a worker requested to work in an area by local residents and a worker commencing work in an area as a result of a new development there, such as the declaration of a Housing Action Area or the announcement of motorway plans, which is going to be important to local people.

Employer's Mandate It is common for teams of social workers or community workers to have no choice about the area to be worked in. The worker or team is appointed following a decision by the agency to place its resources in a particular patch. A local authority will agree to having a project located in one part of its area of responsibility; it then has to decide in which ward, or combination of two wards, the project will be placed. Similarly, a neighbourhood worker may be employed by a local authority to work, for example, on a particular housing estate; quite soon she will have to choose the most appropriate focus on the estate. This could be by area or by group.

When a worker is uncertain as to either the exact territory she will concentrate on out of the wider area or set of issues, a familiar technique is to provide information and advice services as a way of becoming established or recognised: we discuss these in Chapter 6. This form of obtaining entry to a community will reduce the amount of time a worker has to put into meeting and talking with members of community groups, voluntary organisa- tions, churches, and so on. Foster, writing about the beginnings of the North Tyneside CDP, describes how council tenants had been expecting the local authority housing department to establish an office on the estate to provide information about modernisation plans:

> When the project office opened on the estate the general view of the tenants was that the council had decided to play fair and had established a housing unit on the estate from which tenants could get the information they wanted. In fact, the council had established a separate housing office on the estate, but tenants tended to regard the project as this, and largely ignored the official office. (1975)

The project's policy of using its offices as an information centre meant that the team were able to make contact with an increasing number of local people. They combined this with talking to as many people as possible in order to identify the main issues in the area:

> It was in the shops, launderettes, clubs and pubs that issues were raised and information and ideas shared. These are the political meetings and exchanges that take place every day in working class areas. (1975)

It is often neither feasible nor desirable for a worker to offer advice services in order to obtain a more accurate understanding of why she has been appointed to work in a particular neighbourhood and to begin to obtain a mandate from the community. Her chief interest at this stage will be in meeting leaders of groups and organisations. The aim will be to make herself known to them and to begin to build up a picture in her mind of the area's needs and resources, its problems and its potential. She will want to identify informal networks and their leaders, in addition to established groups and organisations.

Request From Local People A few years ago considerable attention was given to a High Court decision in favour of a residents' group in Salford which forced the local authority to keep housing scheduled for demolition in a reasonable state of repair. This example of community action illustrates the situation where a community group asks for support of a worker. The Salford group had approached the regional Shelter office, which agreed that two of its staff would help the group. It was a contractual agreement, whereby the group was clear about its objectives and the workers knew what their task was. In a similar vein, Goetschius describes how London Council of Social Service fieldworkers in the 1950s had an agreed policy that 'Advice should only be given on the invitation of the tenants' committee or of a member or members acting on behalf of the committee' (1969).

In terms of the worker negotiating his or her entry, the parameters are more obvious when a clear request has been made by local people than they are normally. This should not imply, however, a diminution of its importance in the neighbourhood work process. However exact a request or 'contract' may be, a worker has always to win the confidence and trust of local people as well as become known by a range of other key actors.

There are several models of requests made by a community group, or federation of groups, for a neighbourhood worker, and it would be wrong to equate the ability of a community group to request the support of a worker with militancy by a group. For example, sometimes a worker has run down his involvement with a group but has remained available to help it on specific issues if requested. In this case the work of gaining recognition from the group and of ensuring that his or her role is clear can to all intents and purposes be short-circuited: he or she may simply have to re-negotiate entry to the group, especially if its membership has changed significantly.

A forthright exponent of the need for the neighbourhood worker to negotiate entry only when his or her expertise has been requested by local people is Alinsky (1971).

A Potential Issue   A commonplace characterisation of community work is its need to be opportunistic, to 'sense the moment' at the right time. In terms of negotiating entry, two types can be identified. On the one hand, there is the community worker who has become very well informed about, say, one local authority area, although he or she is not involved in neighbourhood work there. She has up-to-date statistics and her contacts in different parts of the local authority structure enable her to be fully aware of future plans or of possible changes to existing plans – the imminent declaration of a Housing Action Area would be an example. The worker becomes part of several key networks, which enables her to piece together information. As a result, she becomes a valuable resource both to community groups, because she is in a position to anticipate events and to supply crucial information.

In this sense we are referring to a strategy which arises at the local level as a result of accurate information received by a worker about a potential issue. The ticket, as it were, with which the worker goes in is her prior knowledge of impending action which will affect a neighbourhood, combined with a hunch that such knowledge will be sufficient to bring about organisation within the community. An example of workers using this approach to facilitate their legitimacy in a community is provided in the study by Wates (1976) of competing plans for a residential square. Its essence seems to lie in the combination of research or investigation of facts about a neighbourhood which have not been made public, along with an instinctive feel for the issue or issues which will mobilise people into some form of collective action or rekindle a dormant group.

The second type of situation which opens the way for a worker can be identified as operating at more than one level. Often it arises out of a major external threat to a neighbourhood the entire responsibility for which cannot be put down to only one agency. Benington (1975) has described how he was able to draw upon data collected by the Community Development Project team for helping the formation of a group in the area where he himself lived. Local grievances were already complex: rumours about roads and redevelopment plans; vandalism and nuisance from the football ground; proposed expansion plans by the football club; the inadequate play facilities. The combination of his involvement

46

in community work as a local resident and as a member of the CDP team sometimes led to confusion, but from the beginning he and a CDP colleague were able to make 'some distinctive contribution' to the local committee's work because of the team's specific technical skills. A major and complex redevelopment plan, such as that for London's docklands, will often provide the opportunity for a team to establish itself in an area because it can demonstrate a knowledge of complex issues which threaten the future living-patterns of local people.

The difference between the two types which we have identified is essentially that between impending changes which originate and take place within a local environment and which a worker who is skilled at recognising early signs of planned change can communicate to other workers; and changes which come from outside an area and which are invariably complex and daunting for local people who will be affected by them. In both cases, the worker openly makes use of his or her prior information to move into a position of being accepted by local people as an organiser with something important to offer. If the worker can show why it is important, she will have begun the process of winning recognition and legitimacy.

In suggesting how workers will need to draw on knowledge and skills to become recognised by existing community groups, we think that they will concentrate on meeting community leaders and influential people. Clearly they should evaluate the viewpoints of such people critically, and it will be essential later on to check out information provided by different individuals. But at this stage they are interested in achieving a broad scan of existing groups and organisations in order to obtain from them little more than an acknowledgement of their future role. There is, as yet *no commitment to action*. Sometimes it is hard to distinguish this kind of early work from social interaction between the worker and community leaders, and the receptivity and hospitality of the latter will sometimes add to the blurring of the difference.

Finally, by thoughtful preparation of the way into a community, workers will gain an important element of confidence. As well as creating a breathing space for themselves before taking on commitments, they also know that they are laying strong foundations for later work. This is important for the inner strengths of workers as well as for the work itself:

Getting started on a new job, perhaps in an unfamiliar community, is one of the most difficult – and most exciting – parts of community organising and social planning. Getting one's bearings before being thrown into the full responsibilities of a job should be a top priority for the organiser or planner beginning work in a new neighbourhood or community. (Cox *et al.*, 1977)

Getting one's bearings, finding one's way around groups, networks and community organisations, is inseparable from obtaining an initial mandate from the community.

Agencies

After discussion with officers from Middlesbrough Borough Council an inter-departmental group of officers was established to look in detail at facilities provided on the estate. At an initial meeting held in Middlesbrough Town Hall attended by representatives of Middlesbrough Planning, Housing and Recreation and Amenities Departments and Cleveland Police, Education Department and the Social Services Department, it was agreed to establish the Brambles Farm Community Project. The Project Group was to consist of representatives of all agencies working on the estate and meetings were to be convened by the Social Services Department. It was felt appropriate that all meetings should take place on the estate.

This extract from a Cleveland council report (1978) gives a hint of the kind of work frequently undertaken by neighbourhood workers in the initial phase of a project. In this case it had been the neighbourhood worker who had prepared a report on East Middlesbrough which identified the particular estate for further study, and it was the worker who serviced meetings of the project group. The worker's contact with a range of agencies tends to conceal that part of the early neighbourhood work process in which we are at present interested: the task of workers to make themselves and their role known to relevant agencies, as opposed only to asking for their advice or sharing data with them. The distinction is an important one, for it is all too easy for a newly arrived worker to assume either that agencies have prior knowledge of her arrival or that they understand her role. Both are assumptions that an incoming worker cannot afford to make.

Knittle writes succinctly of the risks for future work if threats to other agencies are not minimised through the worker engaging their early co-operation:

> Your actions can mean a loss of power, through resources that might otherwise be available to them or through a shift of allegiance of community leaders and citizens. A new programme might imply that other community agencies have not been 'taking care of business' or that they could have done more. You may be entering subject or geographical areas which they feel are their territory. (1976)

It is relatively easy for an agency or coalition of agencies to sabotage the future work possibilities of a neighbourhood worker before he or she has had time to get established and when the worker has no power base in the community to support her. The job of introducing oneself to other agencies, if it is not seen as a sensible and courteous first move, can certainly be prompted by the need to safeguard one's position. It can also be approached in a more positive spirit: as an opportunity to gain easy access to, and knowledge of, a wide range of agencies, several of which may later on be less willing to receive you so openly as on a first visit. It is politic for workers to aim to introduce themselves to a 'mix' of agency personnel: senior administrators and policy-makers as well as fieldwork staff. They should also seek to obtain a balance, in their schedule of meetings, between professional and political contacts.

It will often be the case that when workers are engaged in these meetings their ability to articulate role and objectives will be most tested. Agencies such as the Department of Health and Social Security, the housing department and the social services department, which will usually have their own stake in the neighbourhood where a worker plans to be, will be anxious to find out about his or her intended programme and methods of work. The worker will need to have arguments ready. What kind of community work – agencies may inquire – does the worker intend to do? What does she hope to achieve? What will the implications of this work be for agencies? Which part of the area exactly does she plan to work in? These, and a host of other questions, can damage or enhance a worker's initial reputation depending on what answers are given. Some of the questions a worker will wish to answer as fully as possible, while with others – such as the exact location of the work – a worker will want to hold her options open.

At the same time as gleaning information from these agency contacts and explaining their role, workers are engaged in securing explicit recognition from the agencies for the work they are about to begin. It is a transitory relationship between themselves and agencies, whereby they introduce themselves and thereby facilitate their entry into the community. They will include in their introduction other neighbourhood workers and their agencies located in or nearby the community where they plan to work. Such meetings and visits of observation will often have multipurpose functions: neighbourhood workers can offer an incoming worker valuable advice and information about the area as a whole, they can suggest avenues and contacts to avoid or to aim for, they can explain the kind of projects they are working on and suggest further visits, and they may offer the worker the chance of meeting some of them regularly as a support group.

The Worker's Agency

It may seem self-evident that making oneself known to one's own agency is an early priority for the neighbourhood worker. We saw, however, in the example of the FSU worker quoted at the beginning of this chapter, how easy it is for this task to be pushed to one side by the pressures to move into a neighbourhood; frequently the latter is equated in practice with an early move away from the worker's agency. Such a move is rarely deliberate: the main arena, after all, where neighbourhood work will be done, beckons and usually the worker's own interest and motivation mean he or she needs no second asking.

A strong argument for ensuring that work is done early on with the worker's own agency is that of helping to guarantee self-survival: meeting those who ultimately hold responsibility for policy in the worker's agency is a necessary precaution. The worker needs to have a clear idea of the boundaries for the work perceived by the employer – even if she may decide to challenge them later on.

Through explanatory discussions with a range of staff in the

50

agency, workers can get themselves known about relatively easily and quickly. This is important in terms of role, making clear the similarities and differences between a neighbourhood work role and those of other workers in the agency. It is important also in terms of establishing future allies or contacts in the agency, in the event of the work having policy implications for the agency as a whole, or if the worker needs help in obtaining resources from the agency for a community group. For these reasons, a worker employed in a large organisation will be wise to introduce himself or herself to the relevant administrative staff as well as fieldworkers, managers and researchers.

One worker, newly appointed to a community work post with an area team of a south London social services department, happened to start on a day when all the area officers of the department were meeting:

> I was introduced to them by the chairman, and before their meeting started I went round all of them asking for their phone numbers and saying I would like to come and talk to them about their work. Most of them seemed amazed that anyone should want to do this. I saw it as a way of getting a collection of views from key staff in the agency, on how things worked and who was who.

This may be an untypical example, and the process of a worker picking up unconnected bits of information about the agency is inevitably much longer and more haphazard. It will also, of course, vary considerably according to the type of agency in which a worker is employed. Someone joining an autonomous community work team, for example, will be in a very different position from a worker located on her own in a large agency such as a planning or education department of a local authority.

It is probably both sound strategy and good sense for workers to make clear early on, by the information sought and the people they wish to meet, that their work brief necessitates their working both across departments in their own agency and with a wide range of organisations at local and, occasionally, national levels. Employers of neighbourhood workers have to be aware of the need for workers to have a high degree of freedom of movement across professional and administrative boundaries, and relatively easy access to a range of individuals and information sources, compared with most other professionals. This can include frequent and direct contact with elected representatives. It is easier if a neighbourhood worker begins by penetrating up and across the organisation, and into other agencies and networks. If this work is postponed the access is likely to be more difficult and the opportunity to attempt it may involve time-consuming negotiations later.

Naturally, at the same time that the worker is winning understanding and recognition of her role among colleagues, she is also finding out useful information about the agency – about its administrative and decision-making structures, about the support a worker is likely to receive from various colleagues and sections of the agency when doing community work, and about the likely support and co-operation he or she can offer them. Knittle lists seven questions a worker will be seeking answers to at this stage:

(1) Why is this agency in the community work business?
(2) To what extent is this agency willing to allow community self-determination?
(3) What degree of autonomy does the community worker have working with this agency?
(4) What population does the agency think should be served by a community work intervention?
(5) Does the agency wish to address itself to a specific problem area in a community?
(6) What strategies would be acceptable/possible with this agency?
(7) What resources are available to the community worker through this agency? (1976)

Inseparable from consideration of such questions is another set of questions which focus on authority and power in the agency. To whom are workers ultimately responsible? What community interests are represented on the decision-making body – racial, ethnic, religious, social class, geographical? What is the connection between the decision-making body and the funding source – identical or separate?

It is doubly important for workers to make themselves known to their agency if community work is a new or recent introduction in the agency. Very often, in this situation, community work has been referred to in very broad terms. It is the worker's task to sharpen up any such generalities and thereby to convey as clear an understanding of his or her role as possible. This may not mean, necessarily, that a worker should hasten to rewrite a job description – although that may be desirable at a later stage.

A worker's insistence on obtaining clear, agreed terms of reference for her work can impress upon agency colleagues the nature and purpose of the work which is about to begin in the community. The terms should be reached by the worker and the agency together. Such an educative task is continuous. It does not stop once the worker is involved in action, for the action may require the worker to influence the agreed terms. The point we are emphasising here is the wisdom of beginning the process as soon as the worker joins an agency.

We have argued that the neighbourhood worker needs to be active in three arenas in the process of negotiating entry to undertake neighbourhood work: existing community groups and organisations, voluntary and statutory agencies with an involvement in the area and the worker's own agency. The insertion of this phase at the beginning of the neighbourhood work process will prolong the total amount of time required by the worker before beginning to form community groups; it will increase the pressures on the worker to act. It involves handling face-to-face situations in the community and consideration of prior decisions and plans before anyone is met.

Despite these real difficulties, we suggest that it is essential for workers to tackle the issues of acquiring information, gaining recognition, self-introduction and introduction of others to which we have referred. In addition to having the functional purpose of facilitating work in the community, negotiating entry will also allow the worker time to match up impressions of the future work environment with his or her own confidence and ability.

Negotiating entry reinforces the need for reflection by workers about their own resources as workers and about the goals or vision they set themselves as they move closer to the action phase of neighbourhood work. They should now be better prepared to move into more systematic gathering of data, and we describe this in the next chapter.

CHAPTER 3

Getting to Know the Neighbourhood

This phase of the work is variously referred to as fact-finding, data collection, assembling a community profile, or carrying out an assessment of community needs and resources. The primary purpose of this work is to assemble knowledge to inform the worker's decisions about what issues, problems, groups or agencies he will work with. This gathering of data is rarely sufficient in itself to produce change, but is a prerequisite for planning a large number of strategies available to neighbourhood workers and community groups.

Several writers have suggested that the activity of fact-finding in a neighbourhood comprises the following features.

(1) It is a specific and systematic activity, that seeks to avoid haphazardness and vagueness. It is informed by purposiveness and is guided by the worker's objectives.
(2) It relates to a defined problem, issue, locality or group, and is directly concerned with the here-and-now situations of community residents.

(3) It is as objective and free from bias and partiality as possible in its goals, methods of collection and analysis. If it is, then workers must expect that sometimes their fact-finding will yield data that conflict with or controvert their own and others' opinions and impressions of the community, and are suggestive of areas of work that commend little priority in terms of their interests and values.

(4) It is carried out with the intention of putting the findings to some use. Data-gathering is not 'pure research' or the basis of a sociological study: the worker does it in order to apply its results to what he or she has to do in the community (see Dunham, 1970; Yang, 1966).

Why Collect Data?

This last point suggests one of the most important reasons why neighbourhood workers need to gather data before rushing into action. Data-gathering promotes planning and rationality, and simultaneously informs and puts a limit on the influence of intuition in the making of decisions. It is desirable that choices about what the worker is going to do, how it will be done and the likely consequences, are based on knowledge about community groups, problems and resources. At the least, the worker will need to know what problems are to be identified in a community, and how they are experienced by local people; and what motivation, skills and resources are to be found in the community for dealing with those problems.

There are a number of other reasons for data-gathering in neighbourhood work. It provides a focused and comfortable way of initiating contacts with local people and service agencies; in respect of the latter, visits to agencies to gather facts and impressions about an area can provide the foundation for future work with, or on, those agencies and their staff. The initial fact-finding phase also provides a baseline for more specific pieces of action research that may occur during the later phases of the life of a community group. For instance, data gathered by the worker may be useful in specific studies of, say, landownership, employment, housing conditions and so forth that a group may need to carry out in order to support its case for particular changes in the allocation of resources. The worker's data bank on the area may also be useful to community groups when they have to prepare applications for grant aid.

In addition, there are a number of administrative issues that confirm the importance of this fact-finding phase. First, the worker has a responsibility to provide a data bank on the community that will inform workers who succeed her when she leaves the agency for a new job. Second, it is largely through access to facts about the community that a worker's supervisor will be able to judge (a) that the worker is operating on the basis of knowledge and not guesswork or prejudice and (b) that there is a fit between the worker's interventions and her original assessment of needs and resources in the community. Thus, adequate data are a prerequisite of adequate monitoring and evaluation of the worker's activities, done by the worker and/or the supervisor. Additionally, the worker's (and supervisor's) familiarity with data about the community may often be useful in justifying and supporting some aspect of her work that has come under criticism. For example, a worker in a northern social services department wrote an article for a local newspaper which described the very poor housing conditions in the town. The chairmen of both the housing and social services committees were annoyed by the article and approached the worker's assistant director. The worker, however, was able to show that the article was based completely on the available census data for the town.

The extent of the data-gathering may range from the kind of reconnaissance studies described by Sanders (1973) that involved four or five workers for only a week to larger-scale assessments of need that can last as long as six to nine months. Each worker must come to a decision about the scope and scale of her fact-finding activities in the light of, first, the range and complexity of issues thought to be associated with the area and, second, her own circumstances. A person, for example, who is an area's first worker may have to spend considerably more time in gathering data than someone who joins a team to replace an outgoing worker. Someone who is replacing a worker will presumably have access to data already gathered and, in addition, may find herself quickly embroiled in action as she takes over the work left by her predecessor.

There are several other factors that will determine workers' commitments to fact-finding, including the kinds of skills they have (or have not) for handling data, and their understanding of what they have found helpful and appropriate in past experience. Likewise, the amount of time and energy given to fact-finding will vary directly with the extent to which they see their approach as rationalist, and inversely where a worker believes in a more intuitive approach. In determining what is the 'right' balance between fact-finding and other early activities such as making relationships with residents and agency colleagues, the worker will also be influenced by an awareness of some of the 'dangers' of fact-finding. In particular, workers may be aware that gathering data can provide an inappropriate retreat from the tasks of engaging with local issues and people.

There are two questions to be asked about data collection: what do I need to know? how do I go about finding it out? The rest of the chapter is organised around these questions.

What Do I Need to Know?

It is possible to specify a range of subjects about which data are sought in neighbourhood work. We have divided this range into six categories only for the purposes of analysis. In practice, they overlap and it may be difficult for the worker to know to which category a piece of information belongs. For example, data on a powerful organisation in a neighbourhood are relevant both to the category called 'organisations' and to that called 'power and leadership'. We suggest that the following scheme be used by workers as a guide or checklist in their data-gathering activities, and not as an analysis to straitjacket their own perceptions of the particular, and unique, community in which they find themselves working. In addition, some data about a neighbourhood may only make sense within an understanding of the dynamics of the whole city or region, and data about these wider areas may also be needed.

The following, then, are the six major topics about which you may want to gather data:

history;
environment;

residents;
organisations;
communications;
power and leadership.

History

Issues and problems of an area are connected to people, organisations and events in its past. Local people are often the best sources of historical data, and contacts with them to learn more about the history of the area may develop to the extent that they become involved in organising around a neighbourhood issue. The need to understand neighbourhood issues within a historical perspective has been under-represented in the community work literature, though there are some impressive exceptions; for example, see Benwell Community Project (1978) and Honor Oak Estate Neighbourhood Association (1977).

Environment

The environment of an area is of interest for two reasons. First, it may contain some of the problems of concern to residents (such as inadequate open space) and around which they may want to organise. Second, it provides the context in which people in the area go about their work and leisure and as such may be an important determinant of their relationships with each other. For example, it is common to find in workers' reports an account of a road or railway line that divides an area in half and hinders people either getting together or using services sited on the 'wrong side of the tracks'.

Environmental data that are relevant for the neighbourhood worker include:

the administrative and natural boundaries of the area;
density of persons per acre;
the provision of public open space;
the siting and effect of road, rail and pedestrian facilities;
the volume and nature of road traffic;
land usage in the area, and the interaction and balance between
  industrial, commercial and residential uses. The presence of

derelict and undeveloped sites and buildings will also be something to be noted. Besides their impact on the environment, they may later prove to be a useful resource;

the extent and nature of recreational facilities;

the design and layout of streets and estates, and the way in which they affect residential life;

the extent and content of residents' own destructive and creative attempts at changing the environment through activities like vandalism, graffiti, murals and fly-posting.

The Residents

Data on the people who live in an area are naturally among the most essential for a worker to collect. They are needed not only to understand the nature of the community in which the person is to work but also because some of this data, such as occupation and country of birth, may indicate sites of disadvantage. Data about residents may be usefully classified as follows:

Basic Information This is data about the demographic, housing, employment and general well-being of the people in the area. It includes the following information.

Population: population size and mobility; age and sex of population; country of birth; car ownership; number, size and types of households; socio-economic groups in the population; marital status; educational qualifications.

Housing: overcrowding; tenure; households with and without basic amenities like a bath, WC and hot water supply; the number of dwellings that are occupied, shared and vacant.

Employment: number of employed and unemployed by age and sex; types of jobs held by residents; numbers of women in full- or part-time work; number of people travelling into and out of the area for work; and hours of work of all women, married women and women with children under 5.

These data on population, housing and employment are

obtainable from the census. There are some excellent guides on how to use census material that indicate the benefits and limitations of the census as a source of information (see, for example, Glampson *et al.*, 1975, and Shelter Community Action Team, n.d.). One advantage of the census to the neighbourhood worker is that it provides basic data on residents for each size of area in which the worker may be interested. *National Tables* give figures for areas such as regions, sub-regions, cities, countries, boroughs, new towns and rural districts; *County Reports* for counties, local authority areas, new towns and conurbations; and *Ward Library Tabulations* for ennumeration districts, wards and parishes. It must be remembered, however, that census data can often be out of date, particularly in redevelopment areas.

Additional sources of data on population, h using and employment may also be available in some authorities. For example, some of this data may be culled from the records of a housing department; or an authority may have carried out its own survey of housing conditions in its area.

Social Welfare Data   There is a potentially large amount of data that the neighbourhood worker can use to make an assessment of the general welfare of a community. The sources for this data, and the kinds of information that are available, are described in the pamphlet by Glampson *et al.* (1975). Such data include free school meals; essential clothing allowance; school non-attendance; juvenile first offenders; still births and infant mortality; electricity and gas meter disconnections; social services caseloads and referrals; homelessness; supplementary benefits.

There are a number of difficulties in using such data, and these are discussed by Glampson *et al.*; much of this information is actually about the provision of services in a community and should not be taken on its own to indicate need. Second, the ease of access to this data will vary; information on, for example, supplementary benefits is often particularly difficult to acquire.

Perceptions of the Area   The neighbourhood worker will want to know residents' perceptions of the boundaries of the area, and what they see to be its good and bad characteristics as a place in which to live and work. In particular, the worker will want information on what residents perceive as the problems, issues and resources in the area, and their ideas about the causes of such problems. There will also be interest in residents' attitudes to the various sections and groups that make up the community; and towards service agencies and people like local councillors.

Community Networks Residents will be part of (or perhaps not part of) a network of relationships and contacts within their area. The network will comprise relationships with family, neighbours and friends. The worker needs to understand the extent and functions of these networks, not least because they will be an important part of the support and strengths in a community; a useful resource to developing this understanding are the various sociological studies carried out in communities in this country and the United States. There is also a helpful discussion in Rachelle and Donald Warren's book about types of neighbourhood networks and leadership, and how the neighbourhood worker must understand and use them (1977). Ilys Booker has also suggested that study of these networks of relationship reveal to the worker the people in the community who take on the 'classic roles':

> The worker gradually becomes aware of these group relation-ships and begins to discover that there are some people with specific roles. There are those who represent the social norms and who are therefore reference points in the value system. There are the pace-setters, the critics, the innovators, the reactionaries. In fact, a whole series of classic roles exists. It is these clusters of relationships and their satellites which form the fundamental neighbourhood network which is indispensable to the development worker. (Quoted in Mitton and Morrison, 1972)

Community networks are also of interest to the worker because they will have an influence on his or her work in helping residents organise as a group. Such factors as the dissemination of news and gossip about an issue, the recruitment of group members, and the extent to which the worker is perceived as an outsider will each be partly determined by the nature of community relationships.

Values and Traditions Adequate knowledge about values and traditions is something the worker can hope to acquire only after working in an area for a period of time. Yet he or she has to acquire some understanding of the diversity or nuances of community norms in the early stages of work, not least because decisions must be guided in the light of what are understood to be important values in the community. At the very least, the worker will want to avoid doing things that offend or flout conventions and values in the area. Alinsky has cautioned that workers respect a neighbourhood's norms about dress, language and life-style (1971). The community worker risks alienating people if he knowingly acts outside the standards for what is considered 'proper behaviour' in the neighbourhood.

One of the important tasks when a worker leaves a neighbour-hood is to acquaint his successor with people's expectations about behaviour. For example, a community worker coming new into an on-going project wrote:

> It has already become clear to me that there are significant 'divisions' between various estates in the neighbourhood, and that Dunstable Court (homeless families block) is looked down upon by the rest of the blocks, even by the people in the tenements. George (the out-going worker) warned me about the problems of using the Bull and Plough pub: he said that although it is used by Blackmills Tenants' Association, many of the people in the area think it is not a very respectable place to be in.

The kind of information the worker will be looking for in this phase of the work will largely be concerned with:

Norms that govern social interation and participation in the area, particularly the neighbourhood. For example, a worker was disappointed when few tenants turned up to a meeting in a tenant's flat. He later found out that people in the block were very circumspect about visiting each other's flats, and it was not considered 'to be the done thing'. Second, the worker who wrote about Dunstable Court (above) tried to organise a meeting of local groups to discuss a summer playscheme. There was little interest in the meeting, largely because he had underestimated the strength of feeling against Dunstable Court; the other residents did not want to mix with them at a meeting.
Norms that determine people's attitudes to organising as a group

and taking action to achieve some change. Particularly important are the norms that influence the taking up and exercise of
leadership and authority. Of particular interest may be the
attitudes of men to the involvement of women in neighbourhood work.

Organisations

The first difficulty that we encounter in gathering information
about organisations in an area is that there are invariably a great
number of them, with a diversity of goals, roles and operating
procedures. The neighbourhood worker must first decide on some
way of conceptualising this organisational environment so as to
provide a guide for the arrangement and classification of data.
One way of presenting this material is simply to make a list of
organisations, using a mixture of type and function to decide upon
the headings for this list. This method is illustrated below in
describing the range of organisations that the worker will seek
information about.

Local and Central Government This includes departments
concerned with education, health, planning, social services,
probation and after-care, housing and supplementary benefits.
Information will be needed in each aspect of each department's
work. Education, for example, will need to be looked at in terms
of schools, higher, further and adult education and youth
provision. For each organisation/department the worker will seek
to know:

  the nature and extent of its services;
  its structures, goals, policies, funding and staffing arrangements;
  its impact upon, and intentions for, the community;
  the nature of its relationships and communications with the
    community, and with other organisations;
  what resources it has that may be of use to community groups.

Economic Activities The worker will need to know about the
production and distribution of goods and services in the
community. He or she will want to know not only where people
work (which may be outside the community) but also the range

and importance of industrial, commercial, trade and occupational activities in the area. A worker may try to assess the area's economic base according to whether it is, for instance, manufacturing, industrial, commercial or recreational. He or she may need to construct a history and profile of major employers in the area. Information about transport facilities and retail and wholesale services like shops, pubs, cafes and so on, is also useful.

Other information needed would include that on land usage and zoning and how vulnerable the area is to redevelopment; the balance between private and public industries; and the character of the private rented housing stock, and the renting and management policies of its owners. The worker may want to make an assessment of:

the long-term security and stability of the area's economy, taking into account factors like the narrowness or breadth of its economic base;
the relationship between the economic structure and the social conditions and fabric of the community.

Religious Organisations   The worker will examine these organisations to determine both what they contribute to the life of the area and the nature of any resources (such as a meeting place and duplicating facilities) they may have that would be useful to community groups. The presence and role of such organisations is often a crucial factor in trying to work with ethnic minority groups.

Associations   Most areas have a number of associations/groups pursuing a variety of goals with membership open to the public or certain sections of it. The minimum data that the worker will require about associations are the names and addresses of officers, and any paid staff; time and place of meetings; aims, functions and activities, numbers of members and their characteristics in terms of age, sex, class, income and residence; and an association's resources and facilities.

Voluntary Organisations   The worker will require similar information about voluntary agencies in the area, such as councils of social service, community relations councils and organisations serving particular groups like the aged. These organisations are of particular importance to the worker because:

they are a source of information about the area;
they are potential participants with the worker in dealing with some community issues at a policy level;
they are a possible target of the worker's or a community group's activities where it is seen as desirable to influence the functioning and services of the organisation;
they are a source of resources and facilities for community groups.

Communications

It is central to the neighbourhood worker's task to understand how ideas, information and news are disseminated within the area. The worker wants to know, too, the most effective ways of communicating with key people in the area, whether residents or those in service agencies. It is useful to know which instruments and channels of communication carry weight amongst particular sections of the community and help to shape and change public opinion.

The means of communication in an area will range from informal, verbal contacts, on the one hand, to written, mass-distributed products like newspapers on the other. The neighbourhood worker will need to study fly-posting, leaflets, tenants' newsletters, the house magazines of service organisations, television and radio. As far as newspapers are concerned, the worker may find a range of products, including those of action groups, the alternative press and large-circulation local newspapers.

When a worker is studying newspapers in order to understand the nature of the communications network in an area, questions have to be asked that are different from those used when studying a paper in order to gain information about a locality. R. L. Warren has provided a helpful list of these questions (1955). Such an analysis of newspapers, together with contacts with individual reporters and feature writers, will help to indicate which newspapers will sympathetically report the activities of a community group.

Power and Leadership

By the time the neighbourhood worker has gathered information on the residents, organisations and communications of an area, she will have already amassed a good deal of knowledge about how power, leadership and influence are exercised within the community. Therefore most of the work in this aspect of data collection involves abstracting and synthesising material already gathered. We suggest that data about an area's power structure may be classified as follows.

Business and Organised Labour   The decisions and ambitions of businessmen and trade unions have a very potent influence on the general growth and development of an area. The worker needs to understand how these two interests influence decision-making in the community; particularly that of councillors and officers in the local authority. Business and industry may exercise power either directly or indirectly through organisations like a chamber of commerce or meetings of business and professional people such as the Rotary Club and Round Table.

Elective Politics   Here the worker will study the role and influence of political parties in the area. She will be interested in the strength of ward membership and the percentage of people turning out to vote at local and national elections. The worker will study the power and influence of particular ward councillors (and of the local Member of Parliament) and assess their contributions to policy-making at 'the town hall'. He or she must understand the power of the party caucus and the basis and extent of the power of committee chairmen in the local authority.

Of particular interest will be the degree of involvement, if any, of the traditional political parties in working with local people on community issues. Community groups have often developed to fill a vacuum created by councillors and ward parties. In Notting Hill, for instance, O'Malley argues that it was:

> because the local Labour Party had not provided a real channel through which people could effectively challenge the controlling class interests of the Council and private capital, that a political vacuum had developed . . . which was a necessary condition for

the growth of a strong political life outside the traditional party structure. (1977)

Some excellent examples of studies of political influence and power are to be found in some of the reports from CDP projects and workers. Another example is provided by workers in Wandsworth who have distributed a pamphlet called *Wandsworth Council and How To Influence It – a Guide for Local Groups*.

Administrative Politics This is a phrase used by Cheetham and Hill (1973) to describe the situation where councillors have given most or all of their responsibilities for decisions to the paid officers of the council. We use the phrase also to refer to the general involvement of professional staff in organisational policy decisions. Such involvement may be accorded to staff on the basis of their professional expertise, or because staff are given autonomy in the running of some aspects of a department's activities. It is important for the worker and groups to understand the interplay between the economic, elected and administrative personnel in an area, and their respective and relative contributions to decision-making. In addition, she must identify those in an organisation who understand the nature of her work and would be sympathetic to the work of community groups. They may eventually provide more than support and feed information to the group. Many community groups fighting planning and redevelopment proposals, for instance, have been helped 'unofficially' by basic-grade staff in planning departments.

Civic Politics This term is used to embrace a great variety of organisations and interests who hold and influence power in a community. It includes professional, cultural and religious organisations; the media; voluntary agencies and societies; community and neighbourhood councils; advisory and management committees attached to social services and housing departments; planning forums; and historical and conservationist societies.

Community Politics This includes groups who consist largely of residents in the community. The groups may be organised on a geographic or interest group basis. Examples are tenants' associations, residents' committees, playground associations and a range of groups formed to take action on some community issue or problem. Community politics also refers to meetings of groups in an area such as ethnic groups, lodges, secret societies and cliques. We also include here the exercise of power and influence by key *individuals* resident in an area, who exercise their influence through an informal network of kin and social relations.

We must stress a number of aspects of this categorisation of power and influence. First, the worker must be alert to the fact that alongside the formal and public power structure there is usually a host of people attempting to influence decisions and events. These 'influentials' may range from the open campaigning of a newspaper or pressure group to the covert lobbying of decision-makers by interested parties. Second, formal power-holders exercise that power not only in ceremonies like committee meetings but also in informal ways and on informal occasions. Third, there is a good deal of interplay and overlap between the categories of power we have described. Many individuals will be involved in business and elective and civic politics. Finally, it would be a mistake to see power structures like a local authority as uniform and coherent systems. Any organisation may be seen to comprise individuals and groups in co-operation and conflict with each other about matters like organisational goals, policies and resources. As such they reveal substantial tensions and rivalries that are there to be exploited by a discerning and skilful community group. It is part of the task of the neighbourhood worker to come to know these organisational 'weaknesses' and also to know to what kinds of pressures and publicity they may be vulnerable.

How Do I Go About Data Collection?

We have indicated that there is a daunting array of data that are germane to the neighbourhood worker in the initial phases of intervention. Not only must time and energy be given to choosing and gathering this data, but the worker will also be involved at this stage in other activities such as settling into the agency and making contacts with people in the community and other agencies. The multiple demands on the worker's time in this phase make it necessary that she comes to the task of data collection with a strategy about what data are needed and how they will be collected. There is little point in workers rushing around gathering facts, figures and opinions in one hectic scramble. There are three useful questions to ask of data: do I *need* them? what do I need them *for*? do I need them *now*? There is the danger that without planning the worker will collect so many data that they overwhelm his physical and intellectual capacity to process them. The best way to collect data is to gather them for the particular purposes at hand, rather than collecting them to store, like a squirrel, for some imagined day in the future when they might turn out to be useful.

We have found it helpful to consider four aspects in thinking about how to collect data. They are:

– deciding which neighbourhood to work in;
– taking a first look at the chosen neighbourhood: the broad-angle scan;
– some key principles in collecting data;
– analysis, interpretation and write-up.

Deciding Which Neighbourhood to Work In

In this phase, the worker only needs data that will help decide in which neighbourhood he or she will work. The worker will collect comparative data and will begin to decide on the boundaries of the area in which to work. A project, for instance, coming into a local authority, will set about comparing different areas in the authority in order to choose into which area it should move. It will then need more data to decide upon a specific neighbourhood in that larger area. Likewise, a worker joining an area social services team will have to gather data about the team's area of service in order to decide which particular neighbourhood to move into. The primary purpose of data collection in this phase, then, is to decide to which neighbourhood the worker will commit his or her resources.

In order to make this decision, the worker has to identify areas that are variously described as being in need, deprived or disadvantaged. The worker does not assume that everybody in such an area is in need but that such areas are likely to contain problems and issues to which community work might properly

69

address itself. Thus the worker needs only those data which *indicate* likely areas of social deprivation and disadvantage. The most useful source for such social indicators is the census, and our suggestion is that in this phase the worker need collect only census data that indicate a real concentration of residents who are disadvantaged in the housing, employment and education markets. Such census data would include information on the proportion of privately rented furnished accommodation; the extent of multi-occupation and overcrowding; the existence or lack of basic housing amenities; rate of unemployment; proportion of men in semi- and unskilled occupations; and educational qualifications. Of course, if other social indicators, such as data on free school meals, are available, then the worker should also make use of them. Two articles which provide an introduction to the concept and uses of social indicators are Edwards (1975) and Hatch and Sherrott (1973).

It must be emphasised that the choice of data from the census will be influenced by the worker's values and mandate. If his or her job is to work with particular groups in the population, such as the young or the elderly, then the worker would obviously use the census to search for areas where such groups are to be found.

Having collected census data on the different areas that are 'competing' for his resources, the neighbourhood worker must then rank them on each of those variables that have been taken from the census and decide which area to work in. The ranking of the areas may indicate which is in greatest need, though often the census figures may only distinguish very different areas, for example, middle-class owner-occupied districts from public housing estates. Indicators from the census will often be of limited value and, as Edwards has pointed out, they 'will be but one of a number of inputs to the decision-making process. They will be weighed against convenience, political expediency and such notions as "balance", and "fairness" ' (1975). For example, a worker may decide not to work in a neighbourhood that is indicated as an area of need if, for example, there are already community work resources to be found in it. The worker's choice between areas will also presumably be influenced by impressions formed when walking about in the areas; by the views and priorities expressed by his or her agency; and by the worker's assessment of the potential for achieving change that exists in different neighbourhoods.

Taking a First Look at the Chosen Neighbourhood: the Broad-Angle Scan

The worker may now be ready to study the neighbourhood through what Etzioni calls a 'broad-angle scan' (1967). The purpose of this scan is to determine the principal features of the neighbourhood, and to direct the worker to those aspects of neighbourhood life and issues that he or she wishes to study in more detail. It is clearly not desirable or feasible for the worker to examine exhaustively every aspect of neighbourhood life; the worker is forced at this early stage of the work to be selective in the data collected. He or she may, of course, be selective by randomly or haphazardly choosing features of the neighbourhood to study, but we suggest that a broad-angle scan provides a more reliable and perhaps rational form of guidance as to what aspects of the community should be researched in depth. The broad-angle scan will throw up a series of:

issues (e.g. housing, play, unemployment, traffic, loneliness, neighbourhood care);

groups (e.g. claimants, handicapped, squatters, homeless, elderly);

territories (e.g. particular housing estates or streets);

agencies, organisations and policies; or

existing community groups

that the worker can then decide to investigate further. In addition the broad-angle scan will give to the worker the 'feel' of the neighbourhood, and an overview of its characteristics, both of which are essential to the collection and analysis of data about specific parts or aspects of the neighbourhood.

Before we continue, we offer some words of caution and support that should be borne in mind when reading the rest of this chapter. The emphasis and detail of our discussion of data collection may lead workers and students to spend too much time on it, or even to give up, feeling that they are not adequately prepared for the job. We have tried to be thorough and detailed in our presentation in order to provide a guide as to what *might* be done; it is not our intention to suggest that every worker should collect every kind of data to which we refer. With these words of qualification, we suggest that the broad-angle scan should comprise the following activities.

Analysing the Census   The worker should use the census to acquire basic information about the residents of the area. As was discussed earlier, this includes information on age and sex; place of birth; housing tenure and conditions; socio-economic groupings; types of employment and unemployment. This will often be a re-analysis of the census data collected in phase 1.

Street Work   The worker walks the streets and visits the amenities (cafes, pubs, shops, etc.) of the neighbourhood in order to observe and talk with people. He or she must deliberately seek contact with different sections of the population, and begin to understand which people frequent which parts of the neighbourhood, at what times and for what purposes. Through talking with people the worker seeks indications and clues as to how people see the neighbourhood, and what they perceive as its strengths and weaknesses, issues and problems. The worker also wants to know how the people themselves divide up the area into its constituent patches – which streets go with which streets to form mini-communities within the neighbourhood. Suggestions that might help the neighbourhood worker to structure his or her street work are to be found in Appendix B of the pamphlet by Glampson *et al* (1975) previously referred to.

Scanning Newspapers   Find out what newspapers and magazines are read in the neighbourhood, and read through a selection of back issues. Another reading task at this stage is to obtain a preliminary grasp of the development of the area by going to the local library and seeing if they have a guide to or history of the neighbourhood.

Using the Worker's own Agency Records   The worker should acquaint himself thoroughly with the records and papers of his predecessor, if any, and also scrutinise agency papers and proposals that led up to his appointment, that perhaps indicate needs and issues in the neighbourhood. Any data of his own agency on the area should be examined – for instance, if the worker is employed in the social services then it would be useful to look at data on the team's caseloads and referrals. Some agencies may have produced community profiles before the advent of the worker, though it is often the case that workers are disappointed by the lack of depth in agency views of neighbourhood issues. Finally, the worker should *talk* with agency colleagues, and understand their perceptions of the neighbourhood.

Getting to Know the Authorities   This involves understanding the structures and major provisions of the local authority. The worker may acquire or assemble a directory of the names and addresses of the local councillors, leading politicians, chairmen and members of the authority's committees, and of its principal professional staff. He or she should also study the agenda and minutes from the council for, say, the past year, looking for items about the neighbourhood, and seek out reports on the neighbourhood that may have been prepared by council departments.

Getting to Know Community Groups   The worker should also get together the names and addresses of the officers of any existing community groups, and try to acquire the newsletters and minutes of these groups and begin to understand a little of their origins and functions.

Finding out who Serves the Neighbourhood   Here the worker wants some initial information on the range of organisations and agencies that are based in, or serve, the neighbourhood. At this stage, this kind of information may be best acquired from colleagues in the worker's agency.

Before beginning these various activities that constitute the broad-angle scan, the worker had best think about how much time and energy they will be given. When he or she has assembled and studied this information, the worker should be ready to move into the next phase, which is that of a more detailed and methodical study. However, it may often be the case that the worker feels that he has collected sufficient data through the broad-angle scan to move into the action stage of work. Or the contacts the worker has made have resulted in specific requests for assistance that he feels cannot be refused or postponed. In either of these cases, the worker may decide to proceed no further with data collection. If this decision is made, the worker has to be as certain as possible that he is not moving too soon, or on the wrong issues, or with the wrong people. If, for example, the worker decides on the basis of impressionistic conversations with people that play is an issue in the area, he ought to be sure that play is indeed a concern in the minds of residents, and not just a bee in the bonnet of those few people talked to. One way of finding out is to 'run with an issue' and see what happens. Another way, and one which helps to diminish the possibility of an early failure marring the worker's attempts to organise within the neighbourhood, is to hold off from action for a little while longer and plan and carry out a more detailed collection of data.

Some Key Principles in Collecting Data

These principles about data collection are that it is comprehensive and detailed, and thorough and systematic in its methods. The worker wants to gather valid and reliable data rather than impressions, which contribute to the worker's decisions about interventions. The worker undertakes these activities by using methods and principles that reduce as far as possible the influence of chance, bias and subjectivity on his or her findings. That is, the worker attempts to provide valid and reliable data by (a) using methods of investigation that are commonly associated with social research, such as the survey; and (b) using those methods with due attention to, and understanding of, the principles that inform their use in the field of social research. For example, if the worker carries out a survey, then he must do so with some regard to the principles of survey design and administration. There is also little value in carrying out a survey if insufficient attention has been given to matters like sampling.

The purpose of this section is only to review some of the important methods through which workers may obtain valid and reliable data. Readers must turn to specialised textbooks for further advice on the techniques and principles involved, and we will suggest books that are suitable for this purpose.

Questioning We want to consider the two methods of questioning that seem most common and/or useful to neighbourhood workers. They are the questionnaire and focused interviews.

QUESTIONNAIRES   A questionnaire may be administered by post, by telephone, by asking informants to complete it themselves and calling back to collect it, and by a face-to-face interview. Each way of administering the questionnaire, however, has its own advantages and disadvantages relating to, for example, cost and refusal rate and the worker must assess which method is appropriate to the task in hand. On balance, the personal interview in which the worker asks the questions and records the person's responses is probably the most appropriate for neighbourhood work, not least because it brings the worker into contact with people who might later be involved in the formation and organisation of a group.

Another task for workers is to decide what *type* of questionnaire will be used. Questionnaires vary from being very standardised, on the one hand, to completely unstructured, on the other. We shall discuss the unstructured kind later in looking at the focused interview. In the standardised questionnaire, the interviewers ask the same questions in the same order to everyone who has been selected to be interviewed. The nature of the stimulus to the respondents – the verbal questions – is kept as unvarying as possible. There are two kinds of questions on these questionnaires: the closed or 'fixed-alternative' question in which the respondents are asked to choose between alternative replies; and open questions to which the respondent may reply as he or she wishes, and the interviewer must try to record the response in full.

The following are among the major issues that the worker must consider if he or she decides to become involved in surveys or self-surveys that use a questionnaire. Detailed advice on these aspects of questionnaires should be sought from one of the following textbooks: Hoinville *et al.* (1978); Moser and Kalton (1975). For discussion of the planning and organising of a community study, see R. L. Warren (1965).

The design of the questionnaire.   Thought must be given to the objectives of the survey and the intentions of the worker; the issues or matters that the questionnaire must cover; the form of the questionnaire (how standardised it is to be) and the balance between open and closed questions; its length and the order of questions; and question-wording. The worker must also decide how he or she will approach respondents, particularly how she will explain the purposes and sponsorship of the investigation.

Piloting the questionnaire. It is essential to pilot the proposed questionnaire in order to 'test' it for length, the relevance, wording and sequence of questions, and its overall impact on respondents.

Choosing a sample. Whether or not a sample has to be chosen depends on the size of the group or population in which the worker is interested, and the time, money and help at his or her disposal. The advantage that sampling has over haphazardly picked-out individuals for interviewing is that it allows one to make inferences from the sample about the population from which it has been chosen.

There are different kinds of sampling methods and these are discussed in the books by Hoinville *et al.* and by Moser and Kalton. The three kinds of sample likely to be of most use to neighbourhood workers are the *simple random sample*, the *systematic sample* and the *quota sample*. In the simple random sample each member of the population has an equal and known chance of being selected; the selection is made by assigning a number to each unit of the population from which the sample is to be drawn. Identification of the units that will make up the sample is achieved by a number of techniques, including drawing numbered discs from a bag, the use of random number tables, or a computer.

Systematic sampling involves drawing every nth unit (a person or a household, for example) from a list of those units. Taking every tenth name from an electoral register, or every fifth name from a list of community groups in an area, or taking every third case from a list of an agency's clients, are examples of sampling systematically. Systematic sampling is not strictly random because the people on a list do not have an equal chance of inclusion; the people that fall between the nth persons have no chance of inclusion.

In quota sampling, the interviews are given quotas of people to interview. They are asked to interview so many people according to, for example, different age, sex, class and housing tenure groups. The number of interviews that are to be with men and women, or with different ages, is calculated from available data like the census. For example, if 60 per cent of the residents in a street are female then the worker would ensure that 60 per cent of the people he interviewed were female. An example of the use of quota sampling in community work is contained in the account of the Southwark Community Project (Thomas, 1976, ch. 4). The relative strengths and weaknesses of these three and other methods of sampling are discussed in the textbooks to which we have referred.

Interviewing also poses particular problems for the neighbourhood worker and for members of a community group carrying out a self-survey. On the one hand, they will be interested in building up rapport with residents; on the other, they must guard against their interests, opinions and values about neighbourhood issues influencing and distorting the replies that the respondents offer.

These cautionary words about some aspects of the use of questionnaires serve to indicate that to do a survey or self-survey will require a good deal of study, time and skill. Before embarking on a survey, it is best to make sure that the information that is required is not already available, or cannot be acquired through means other than a questionnaire. The self-survey may be seen to be a more attractive proposition to the worker because it makes use of available resources in the community. But the participation of residents and/or colleagues does not necessarily represent a simple gain in numbers of people and hours. The worker will find that time has to be allocated to:

the recruitment and encouragement of helpers;
work with them to discuss the purposes of data collection, and the design and planning of the methods to be used;
training them in the use of the methods if they are unfamiliar;
supervising their work, and being available for support and discussion when helpers find problems or when their enthusiasm wanes;
the collective analysis, interpretation and presentation of the data that have been assembled.

Additionally, there may be disadvantages to using local people or agency colleagues. Residents may be reluctant to answer questions posed by neighbours; or by, for example, social workers whose involvement in a survey may be misinterpreted. Another argument against self-surveys is that the group which undertakes the work may too easily become the nucleus for a task or issue group that may emerge from the work carried out on the survey.

People may come to expect the self-surveyors to take on the problems and the self-surveyors may not be able, or want, to handle the expectations they generate.

The self-survey has, however, advantages because of the fact that it involves local people. Self-surveys are more oriented to taking action on a particular issue, and are often used to prepare people for collective action by getting them involved in the collection and analysis of information. For a detailed discussion of the pros and cons of self-surveys and for advice on carrying them out the reader is referred to the books by Weiner (1972) and Robertson (1976).

FOCUSED INTERVIEWS These may be seen as less standardised and structured forms of a personal interview using a question-naire. The interviewer has a checklist of questions or issues to raise with the respondent who is allowed to answer them freely. Likewise, the interviewer is free to probe the respondent's replies as seems appropriate, and to add to, and modify, the interview as it proceeds if the respondent raises relevant but unanticipated issues. Such interviews are also focused by virtue of the fact that they are planned. The interviewer (in this case, the neighbourhood worker) must think about how he will present himself and his objectives, and prepare a strategy that specifies what information he wants, how he will ask for it, and what factors will hinder and facilitate the interviewee's co-operativeness.

There seem to be three primary uses to which the focused interview can be put in data collection. First, it helps the worker to understand more thoroughly how local residents perceive and describe the area in which they live. It permits the worker to acquire some understanding of how residents 'name the world'. Second, it provides the main tool for acquiring detailed informa-tion about agencies and organisations operating in the neighbour-hood. The worker carries out a series of focused interviews with agency staff. Discussions of such interviews carried out by CDP research teams are to be found in Hatch *et al.* (1977), and Mackay (1975). Third, the focused interview is useful in acquiring more information about particularly complex aspects of community life. For example, it may be used to build up information about power, leadership and influence in a community, and Sanders has described one way of doing this (1973, ch. 21). Additionally, the worker can interview a range of people in order to understand the different perceptons of an issue in a neighbourhood such as homelessness, unemployment or loneliness.

Before completing this section on questioning it is worth referring briefly to a range of methods of data collection that are generally referred to as 'indirect'. They include the following:

Sentence completion, e.g. 'If there is one change I would bring about in this neighbourhood, it would be . . .'

The projective question, e.g. 'Suppose a Person from Mars came down to this neighbourhood, and you were the first person she saw, and she asked you what kind of neighbourhood this was; what would you tell her?' Another form of the projective question involves asking the respondent about the views of other people, e.g. 'Some people who live in this estate find a lot of faults with it. I wonder if you can guess what they are referring to?' (These examples are based on those used in Selltiz *et al.* 1976.)

Adjective checklist. Respondents are shown a list of varied adjectives that purport to describe the neighbourhood. The respondents are asked to say which they think apply.

Inventories. There are two kinds which seem potentially useful in community work. With the first, respondents are shown a list of problems/needs and asked to indicate the problem(s) that most affect them as residents in the neighbourhood. The second kind of inventory contains a list of general statements (e.g. 'Shopping facilities for old people in this area are poor') and respondents are asked to say whether they are true or false.

Indirect methods such as these originated in clinical and social psychology but they are being used more in community settings, not least by market researchers. We believe they offer a useful alternative to questionnaires to the neighbourhood worker engaged in data collection. Readers who want to learn more about them are referred to the books by Selltiz *et al.* (1976) and Oppenheim (1968).

Observation By this phase of intervention, observing what goes on in the neighbourhood will have become second nature to most workers. But observation can be undertaken in a more systematic fashion, paying more regard to certain principles and care in the collection, recording and analysis of the data obtained. Lambert has written some wise words for community workers about participant observation:

> This research style is probably the most natural for the community worker but properly done it only *seems* like hanging about and doing nothing. It is easy for it to remain on a glib and superficial level. To go beyond, it needs to be rigorously organised and disciplined and, when subject to the critical demands of a research approach, it can yield a breadth and depth of knowledge of great usefulness. (1977)

One of the first decisions for the worker wishing to organise a more systematic form of observation is the degree of participation. At one extreme the worker can be a complete observer with very little interaction with the observed who may not know what the worker is or what his job in the community is; at the other extreme, the worker will be so keen on building up relationships with local residents that he or she maximises participation and attempts to share as many experiences of the observed as possible. This stance may endanger objectivity. As with personal interviews, the worker must strike a balance between satisfying his or her requirements as a community worker and satisfying those as an investigator and collector of information.

One thing is clear, however; the worker will seldom want to be a totally passive observer. It will be found that the degree of participation with those being observed will vary with factors like the length of time the worker has been in the neighbourhood, and the social setting in which the observations are taking place. A more active role is also made likely by the fact that participant observation consists not only of observations but also of questions of, and interviews with, those being observed.

The participant observer's use of questioning is, of course, in accord with the values and principles of questions within community work practice. The use of the question is an important element in practice as described by writers such as Saul Alinsky and T. R. Batten. Ilys Booker has also vividly described the systematic use of questioning:

> One technique used is to ask a great many questions and, when the opportunity presents itself, especially to ask 'Why?'. The

question may produce information or considered and balanced responses. On the other hand, it may produce replies which indicate prejudice, rejection of any possibility of changing the status quo, a lack of orderly thought process or some other conceptual failure. Furthermore, the raising of the question itself often causes people to give further consideration to it and not infrequently results in new awareness. Each event and each encounter is a potential point for discussion about the area, its population, its communal attitudes, its strengths and its defects. In these discussions many opinions and points of view come to light about the self-image of various sections of the community, their images of each other and their views about voluntary agencies and statutory bodies. (Quoted in Mitton and Morrison, 1972)

There are two types of questioning that seem to be part of the participant observer's techniques for gaining data. They have been described by Strauss as the *reportorial* type of question in which respondents are asked informally about the who, what, where, how and why of events, and the *posing* types of questions. Strauss distinguishes between the following types of posing questions:

The challenge or devil's advocate question. The fieldworker deliberately confronts the respondent with the arguments of opponents. The idea is to elicit rhetorical assertation and thus to round out the respondent's position by forcing him to respond to challenge.

The hypothetical question. This kind of question is another technique for rounding out the respondent's thought structure but without accompanying rhetorical heat. The fieldworker poses a number of possible occurrences (e.g. 'What would happen if you stopped paying rent?'). An extended example of both types of posing question is provided by Alinsky (see 1971, pp. 72 ff.).

Posing the ideal. There are two variations on this technique. First, the respondent can be asked to describe the ideal situation. Secondly, while the fieldworker can still pretend to be somewhat naive, he can assert an ideal to see what response is elicited. Happily, what usually happens is that, when the investigator poses an ideal, respondents not only counter with other ideals, but, in the process, tend to point out the shortcomings of reality.

Offering interpretations or testing propositions on respondents. It is sometimes very useful to tell respondents about the propositions that one is beginning to pull together about events interesting to them. If they disagree, they will usually volunteer information to counter a proposition, which may lead the fieldworker into further unanticipated search. If they agree, the tendency is to qualify the proposition: it does not quite meet the case. Again, the fieldworker comes away with additional valuable information. (Taken in full from Strauss *et al.*, 1964, and reprinted in McCall and Simmons, 1969.)

As with other forms of collection, attention has to be paid in participant observation to the design of fieldwork, sampling, entering the fieldwork situation, record-keeping and the interpretation and analysis of data. Recording observations is particularly difficult in participant observation, and most observers have to rely on a combination of memory, symbols and discreetly written notes. Detailed advice on carrying out participant observation is given in the books by Bogdan and Taylor (1975) and McCall and Simmons (1969).

Using Written Materials We have already stressed that the census is likely to prove the most valuable written source of data and we have already indicated what data should be extracted from the census in the broad-angle scan. In this section we wish to deal briefly with three other types of written material.

LOCAL NEWSPAPERS A worker in a neighbourhood may want to undertake a more systematic analysis of the content of local newspapers in order to add to knowledge of felt and expressed needs.

The special technique for analysing the content of the media is called *content analysis*. The first task is to decide which local newspapers to study. It is fortunate that most neighbourhoods are served by only one, at the most two, large-circulation local newspapers, so the worker may decide to study all the local papers read in the neighbourhood. These papers are also likely to be weeklies. The worker may also decide to study the content of newsletters and community newspapers put out by community groups.

It is unlikely that time will be available to study all the issues of local publications, so the worker must prepare a time sample. He or she might, for instance, decide to study all the issues of the local weekly newspaper that have appeared in the last six months, that is, about twenty-six. How many issues to read and analyse will partly be determined by how much time is available, and the worker can clearly choose a larger sample if help is available from local people or agency colleagues. The next step is to determine which parts of the newspaper will be studied – headlines, editorials, features, news, photographs, and so on. Alternatively, the worker may decide to analyse the content of the whole of the newspaper.

The most basic aspect of content analysis is to note the frequency with which certain items appear in the newspapers. So the worker must decide what kinds of items are to be counted. For instance, he or she may prepare a list of categories of need or issues in the neighbourhood such as play, housing, transport, shopping facilities, and so on. The worker will need to be clear what the 'rules' are for classifying an item within one of these categories. He then proceeds methodically to classify newspaper items within these categories, noting the number of appearances of articles, features, editorials, letters, and so on, concerned with one of the categories. When this has been done, the worker is in a position to count up the items found in the categories, and this will give a simple quantitative indication of which issue seems most important (as measured by the frequency of its appearance).

Counting the number of times an issue appears is, of course, a very superficial form of content analysis. If the worker wants to improve on this then he can use refinements like considering the amount of space that is given to various neighbourhood issues by measuring column inches. The findings of a content analysis such as the one described are not unambiguous. The frequency with which issues are mentioned may just as well reflect the editorial policy or interest of the paper as felt and expressed needs in the community. The usefulness of data derived from a content analysis of papers is that they can be added to the worker's store of knowledge about the neighbourhood that has been acquired from a range of other sources.

LOCAL HISTORY SOURCES Having gained some familiarity with the area's history, the worker may now want to extend and deepen this knowledge. The best way to start doing this is to go to the local library. It will contain books, guides, directories and maps about the neighbourhood and its hinterland; it may also possess primary source material like archives and public, family and business records. There will almost certainly be a librarian who will not only advise on primary and secondary sources but may also be a source of information in his or her own right. Some libraries also produce written guides to local history sources that are available. Another useful place to seek information and advice is a local history society.

Most workers will have limited time and interest in understanding the local history so presumably they will need to be selective in what they study. A worker, for instance, might only want to know about the development of a particular trade or industry or geographical patch and this will provide the boundaries for the inquiries. Some may choose to get an all-round appreciation of the neighbourhood's history. In this case, they might confine their study to getting information on the origin and growth of the settlement; changes in population size and structure; housing and living conditions; the economics, occupations, and employment of the neighbourhood; and changes in values and traditions, particularly as they relate to socialisation processes through institutions like the family, education and religion.

Any worker who believes it is important to study primary sources of information needs to be aware that there are, as in all other aspects of data collection, systematic and thorough ways of proceeding. Advice on method in historical research, as well as information on the range of primary sources that are available for the study of the history of a community, is given in the books by Hoskins (1968) and Iredale (1974). Advice on how to write local histories has been provided by Dymond (1981).

AGENCY RECORDS The worker will have examined his or her own agency's records, and will also have used information from a variety of agencies in compiling the social indicators that were used to help in the decision about which neighbourhood to work in. Data from agency records also complements the profiles on agencies' structures, services and policies that the worker constructs from focused interviews with agency staff.

The neighbourhood worker may make a special study of agency records, not just to gain additional information about the agency, but largely to understand more about needs and issues in the neighbourhood. Most central and local government agencies gather data about their service-users and the 'state of the neighbourhood' quite routinely. Such data include, for example, social services case record analyses, health and education statistics, crime records, and so forth. Besides records on their services and users, most agencies also produce reports, minutes, brochures and annual reports.

There are difficulties in using agency data. The geographical areas for which local agencies keep data are very seldom coterminous, and often they are larger than the area or neighbourhood in which the worker is interested. In such cases, the worker may need to seek access to the raw data from which the agency's records have been compiled.

Analysis, Interpretation and Write-up

It is misleading to present analysis, interpretation and write-up as terminal activities in phase 4. They are, and ought to be, on-going activities to which the neighbourhood worker pays attention from the first phase of data collection. Analysis of data must go hand-in-hand with its collection, if only to guide the worker in decisions about further material required. Each phase of the process of data collection should end with a review of the data so far assembled so that they may inform what has to be done in succeeding phases. It is also more efficient and interesting and less error-prone to analyse and write up data as one proceeds, rather than leaving oneself with a large amount of information to wade through at the end of the process of collection.

The analysis and interpretation of quantitative and qualitative data about a local neighbourhood demands of the worker skills and objectivity of a high order. They have been described by one community worker as follows:

> one has to develop the mental skill of overlapping or overlaying perceptions of the area and to combine that with statistical information . . . there's a skill in building profiles and evaluating and assessing the work that needs to be done in terms of locally felt needs . . . there's a skill in acquiring information about political systems, bureaucracies and forces which have an effect on a particular area . . . also there's a skill in applying

information, fitting it and presenting it in ways which will be understood without over-simplifying, of pitching information without distorting it. (Quoted in Thomas and Warburton, 1977)

There are two major aspects of the analysis and interpretation of neighbourhood data. First, the data must be scrutinised in relation to their validity, reliability and relevance. The worker has to decide which data ought to be put aside, and which may be safely and honestly used as a basis for decisions about work. The claims of conflicting or contradictory pieces of information have to be evaluated. Second, the data have to be 'broken up' in order to discern the various issues, trends and relationships that they contain. While the highest possible standards of analysis have to be brought to bear on the data, it is equally important that the worker does not lose sight of the fact that the collection and analysis of data has been undertaken as an aid to action. They must thus be analysed and written up in ways that facilitate decisions that the worker must take about future activities.

Writing up the Data The extent and nature of the report of the data will largely be determined by what the worker plans to do with the report. Writing up one's analysis and conclusions is only part of a total process, and the worker must decide what his or her objectives are in spending time and energy on writing a report. What the worker intends to do with the report, or the kind of action he or she envisages taking when the report has been produced, should determine the kind of report written.

Report writing, like most things, ought to be planned, and one of the key planning questions is: for whom will I be writing this report of my data collection? In other words, who will be the kinds of people to read it? You might expect that the write-up will be read by as diverse an audience as community residents, agency colleagues and managers, elected members and staff in other agencies concerned with the neighbourhood. If this is the case, then the worker must consider two further issues in planning a report:

(1) *Is one report sufficient?* Should I not consider writing a number of reports, each one geared to a particular set of

readers? The worker might consider that a report that is suitable, say, for his or her agency may not be the most appropriate for influencing councillors or for raising awareness among residents about the needs and issues 'uncovered' in the collection of data.

(2) *How do I empathise with my potential readers?* In order to make an impact with the report, the worker must think himself (or herself) into the minds of those for whom he is writing, trying to assess the kind of write-up that best communicates to them. Abrams (1975) has suggested that there are four problems in communication. First, using the *medium* most likely to come to the attention of the people addressed. Thus, video may be a more appropriate medium for local people (and councillors?) than a written report. Second, using *language* which is readable by the people to whom the communication is directed. Third, employing *concepts* that are within the comprehension of the audience. Fourth, convincing the audience that what they have read and intellectually understood is relevant to their needs and purposes. Saul Alinsky has summarised all these prescriptions for effective communication in the phrase 'always communicate within the experience of your audience.'

Besides recognising that there may be a need for varying the medium, style and content of the write-up for each set of readers, there is also the fact that the communication of the products of the data collection may be achieved through different *types* of report. These include the following types:

A data bank	This will comprise the raw material gathered by the worker, including quantitative data and the results of observations, focused interviews and content analyses. This data may have to be consulted by the worker, and other staff and residents, in the future, in order, for instance, to make an application for a grant.
Working papers	Another possibility is to write papers around each of the major issues or

themes that have emerged in collecting data. The worker, for instance, might want to prepare a paper on homelessness; or income maintenance; or about a particular estate or set of streets.

Feed-back papers Papers might be prepared that provide feed-back to those from whom the worker received information or who helped in the collection of data. The feed-back might be about the outcomes of the data collection as a whole, or about the specific interests, services, and so on, of those interviewed.

Popular papers These might include articles for newspapers, tenants' newsletters, broadsheets and leaflets that help to disseminate the findings of the data collection to a wider and lay audience.

Organisational profiles In the course of data collection, much information will have been collected about organisations serving the neighbourhood. This material can be brought together in the form of profiles of the most important organisations, and these may be useful to the worker and community groups in future relations with the organisations.

Survey reports There may be a case for separate reporting of any surveys that have been undertaken during the collection of data, for example, surveys on the needs of the elderly; or the handicapped; or of transport facilities. It may be advisable to deal with these separately because they may be suitable for a distribution that is wider than the neighbourhood or even the particular local authority.

Community profile This is the report in which the worker seeks to present data about the neighbourhood as a whole. It may take one of two forms. First, a limited neighbour-hood analysis of the kind described by Baldock which 'is roughly equivalent to an "initial diagnosis" document in case-work' (1974). It is a selective presenta-tion of the data, and the selection is made on the basis of some of the decisions the worker has already made about what his or her future activities are likely to be. It presents the data that provide the evidence either for the work-er's preferred analysis of issues in the neighbourhood or for decisions taken about possible action.

The second form of community profile is more comprehensive. It seeks to bring together in an ordered manner all of the data that the worker has gleaned about the neighbourhood. As such, it may also be widely used as a sourcebook of data, together with the data bank of the raw material.

We do not suggest that it is necessary for every neighbourhood worker to prepare all of these kinds of report of data collection. To do so would be to give to data collection a proportion of field time that may not be justified. The point is that workers are aware that there are a variety of forms of writing up their data, and they should choose those that seem most appropriate in the light of the data and the worker's own circumstances. Nor do we want to suggest that the writing-up of data will come to an end at the termination of data collection. There will be many occasions when both workers and groups will need to refer to the data and write it up for some special purpose. In particular, the data are likely to be used to support applications for funds and other resources. The writing of proposals for grant aid, whether to one's own authority, central government or trusts, is a skilled activity in its own right, about which neighbourhood workers and groups should seek advice before putting pen to paper. The following are useful reading in this respect: Ecklein and Lauffer (1972) and Glampson et al. (1975).

The Art of Writing Reports

We want to conclude this section by reviewing a few points about the skills and knowledge involved in writing reports of the kind we have discussed so far. Most workers will come to their first jobs with little or no experience of report writing. What writing they will have done will have been confined to school and college papers, though some will have written, or participated in the preparation of, research reports.

For most workers, then, skill in report writing is something to be learnt on the job, and there are some very helpful guides in this task (Mitchell, 1974). Perhaps the most essential aspect of communicating effectively through reports is that of the planning and layout of the report. All too often communication is impaired by the failure to arrange the content of the report in an orderly and logical manner. We find reports without titles, contents list or page numbering; we often fail to assimilate the contents of a report because the writer has not provided an abstract or a summary. The provision of a summary is vital if the report is to be read by busy people who in the course of their work have also to read a lot of other written material.

The parts of the report should be clearly identified, as should headings and subheadings. The margins and space between lines should be generous to make it easier for readers to read and to make notes. Other helpful hints on clear expression are provided by Mitchell, such as the use of short sentences and paragraphs, avoidance of double negatives, the use of the active not passive tense and the sparing use of adjectives and adverbs. The effective presentation of statistics presents particular problems, especially if lay readers are involved; the imaginative use of maps, pie charts, graphs and histograms are to be preferred to tables or figures.

Conclusions

While this chapter has been concerned with the collection of a wide variety of data about a neighbourhood, it has tended to emphasise the collection of data that indicate the existence and extent of issues and problems. But the worker will also be collecting information about the resources and strengths of an area, and some assessment of these must also feature in a written analysis of the data he has collected. Neighbourhood workers have also used several different methods of classifying information about resources and making it available to groups and to agency colleagues. These include plotting resources on maps, and the use of resource directories and card index systems.

There are two other important activities that neighbourhood workers are involved in simultaneously with data collection: these are making contacts with local people and developing working relations with colleagues and managers in their own agency. Both these activities can lead to early requests for help, or the involvement of the worker in agency activities such as membership of an agency working party. Workers have thus to manage their time and commitment in data collection in relation to these other demands made upon them. Additionally, the phases of data collection and making contacts are frequently described by neighbourhood workers as amongst the most stressful and lonely in the whole process of community work. Stress, uncertainty and anxiety about the real or imagined expectations of colleagues and residents about community work serve to constrain the time and energies available for data collection.

We end this chapter by repeating a point we have made several times before: data collection is not a research project to be pursued for its own sake. It is done in neighbourhood work in order to facilitate planning and action. Data collection, analysis, planning and action are the key and interlocking ingredients of a systematic approach in neighbourhood work. At the outcome of data collection, the worker should be able to prepare an options paper that specifies the actions that might be taken in the light of identified issues and resources. The preparation of a plan of intervention is the subject of the next chapter.

CHAPTER 4

What Next? Needs, Goals and Roles

Planning is a purposeful and conscious act of anticipation through which we attempt to envisage the future. Through planning we seek to attain future states seen as desirable, and to avoid those that we see as undesirable. Planning may also be used to maintain all or some aspects of the status quo. It is through planning our activities that we try to reduce our reliance on chance and accidents in attaining our goals. In this way, we plan in order to bring more certainty and predictability to our future activities and, in addition, to make them more certain and predictable to those who work with us. It is through planning, too, that we are able to state goals and targets and be in a position to monitor progress in achieving those goals.

Thinking about things in our heads before we rush into action does not mean that workers should, or will be able to, stick rigidly to plans once they have been conceived. Workers must be prepared, first, to modify their intentions in the light of changing circumstances in the community and in the organisations and groups that affect their work, and, secondly, to be alert to chance events in the turbulence within and around a community group.

We suggest that there are four major tasks for the worker to accomplish in deciding what to do next. They are:

assessing the nature of problems and issues;
setting goals and priorities;
deciding on role predisposition;
specification of next moves.

We shall look at each of these in turn.

Assessing the Nature of Problems and Issues

As a result of collecting and assessing data, the worker will be aware of those factors in the neighbourhood that are seen by residents and professionals (and by himself) as concerns, issues or problems. This work will have helped him to discover the issues of greatest salience for people. In effect, the worker will draw up a list of such problems and issues – playspace, house-bound mothers, bad housing, inadequate pedestrian crossings, poor shopping facilities, and so on – and a next step will be better to understand these issues through a *problem analysis*.

Such an analysis of problems requires the worker to define the problem and spell out its key dimensions; to understand how the problem is defined and labelled (e.g. by residents and elected members); to determine the size and scope of the problem; and to gather evidence, theories and hypotheses that might help to explain the causes and persistence of the problem.

The assessment and analysis of problems and issues may, for the purposes of discussing them here, be separated out into the following major components (we have been helped in writing this section by Zweig and Morris, 1975, Stein and Sarnoff, 1964, and Cartwright, 1973).

Description of the Problem

The worker's first task in problem analysis is to try to understand how the issues that have been 'discovered' are described by the variety of people with whom he has been in contact. We suggest here that descriptions of problems are different from definitions of problems (to be discussed next) and the worker must try to understand the ideas, concepts, words, phrases, and so on, that people use in their everyday descriptions of the problem. In particular, the worker must attend to the everyday descriptions that local residents use, and be alert to the content and nuances of the vocabularies in the neighbourhood used to 'name the world' and its problematic features. Building up knowledge of these descriptions is part of the continuing process of increasing one's familiarity with a neighbourhood and identification with its inhabitants. There seem to be three important reasons why the neighbourhood worker should attune himself to people's problem descriptions.

First, in order to communicate it is necessary, as Alinsky has emphasised, to talk within, and not go outside, people's experience. The worker is more likely to stay within their experience if he is familiar with the way in which they are accustomed to think about and describe problems that they face. Alinsky has also pointed out that familiarity with people's experience 'not only serves communication but it strengthens the personal identification of the organiser with the others, and facilitates further communication'.

Second, the worker needs to empathise with local people, to put herself in their shoes, and try to understand the problems *as they experience them*. Such empathising is a sound counter-weight to any inclination on the part of the worker to 'intellectualise' residents' problems, or to attribute to them perceptions of a problem that are largely her own.

Third, the language that residents use to describe problems may provide an indication to the worker of their motivation to do something about those problems. Language can be a significant clue both to the extent to which people are critically reflecting on the problematic features of their situation, and of the degree to which people feel able enough to challenge the forces that they see as creating those problems. Descriptive language thus points to the inner political world of community residents, and may be suggestive of the extent of the feelings of powerlessness, alienation, resignation and apathy. Norman Dennis has provided some examples of residents' attitudes to demolition of their homes, couched in language that leaves the impression 'that it would be as meaningful to talk about doing something to prevent the ebb and flow of the tides'. Their comments were:

I went to the Town Hall about it, but they want it, so that's the end of it. There's nothing more we can do. It seems as if they are stuck on it, they said word had come from London that they had to come down.

The Corporation takes no notice of the opinion of people like us. They'd ask the directors of Joblings, but not us.

We wouldn't stand a chance. It's up to them with their own houses to see about it. They wouldn't ask me nothing. I'm just a tenant.

You could sign a petition, but what's the use? You can't go up against the Law. (1970)

Definition of the Problem

The worker's task here is to extend his or her understanding of the key historical and operational dimensions of the problem or problems. While a major question in approaching the first stage of *describing the problem* is 'how do people *experience* this problem?', the question now is 'how is this state of affairs described by residents, *defined* as a problem, by whom, and why?'.

We have here introduced the distinction between a state of affairs or a situation, and a problem. This distinction is important because people may describe a state of affairs (such as 'My flat has no inside WC or bath') without also perceiving and defining it as a problem. States of affairs become problems only through a process of definition and labelling (usually because the states of affairs threaten important local or national values); the worker must not assume that because states of affairs in the neighbourhood are defined as problematic by himself and other professionals they are necessarily seen as such by residents. A worker may be appalled by the housing conditions in a tenement block and also puzzled that tenants do not, or prefer not, to define the conditions as problematic. The tenants may be aware primarily only of the advantages of their tenement (e.g. cheap, centre-city living), or they may, as an underclass, be resigned to low expectations and few ambitions about their housing rights and conditions. In this latter situation, of course, the neighbourhood worker may find that a prerequisite of organising the tenants around the issue of their housing is that he or she first raises the level of their consciousness about their situation.

Thus, the worker wants to know, first, do residents define states of affairs as problematic? If so, how and why are they so defined? Second, if these states of affairs are defined as problematic in the wider society, what are the key historical, conceptual and operational features of the problem definitions? As far as the historical and conceptual features are concerned, the worker who, for example, is working with the problem of housing, will want to understand better what 'over-crowding' and other key concepts mean. A worker alerted to the problems described by, say, mothers in a high-rise block will want to know what 'isolation' or 'privatisation' means. The operational features of a problem would include analysis of the laws and conventions pertinent to the problem, and the administrative/political structures that take decisions in respect of that problem.

The worker may not, of course, have the knowledge or the previous experience to be able to explore the definitions of all the problems encountered in work. No person can be expected to be competent in all aspects of the diversity of problems generated in inner city areas – in the fields, for example, of housing, public health, employment, welfare rights, transport, planning and education. Most workers will have to 'mug up' on problems as they are thrown up by the community, and Patrick Harris has pointed to the important role of the agency supervisor in helping the worker find the appropriate experts with whom to discuss the particular problem area (1977).

There are, of course, limits to the thoroughness with which the worker can explore the definitions of the particular problem. Limits are set by scarcity of time and energy, the absence of available or understandable expert opinion and the pressing need for action on the problem or issue.

The Extent of the Problem

An analysis of a problem would be incomplete without an understanding of its size, scope and effects, and the following seem to be the primary points for consideration.

What are the numbers of people affected by the problem? How many are affected directly, and how many are affected indirectly or peripherally?

In what ways does the problem affect the people involved? How does it influence and determine the various aspects of their lives?

How long has this situation lasted, and how long has it been experienced as a problem by the people? For how long will it persist if the people do not do something about it themselves?

What is the geographical locus of the problem, that is, in what parts of the neighbourhood/estate/block, etc. is the problem to be found?

What social values are threatened by the existence of the problem (and led to a state of affairs being labelled as problematic) and which values and norms in the neighbourhood support, and which oppose, the existence of the problem or problems; that is, what individuals and sections of the community stand to gain, and which stand to lose, by attempts to ameliorate or eliminate the problem?

Arriving at an idea of the extent of a problem, however, is not just a matter of aggregating quantitative data; it also involves assessing qualitative data about how people experience the problem.

The Origins and Dynamic of the Problem

Having defined the nature and extent of the problem, the worker will need also to understand how that problem has come about, to ask questions about its origins, and to think about factors that he believes are responsible for causing, perpetuating and aggravating the problem. In other words, the worker will have hypotheses about causation that are an integral element of problem assessment because they will presumably have an important bearing on the kinds of 'solutions' the worker will come up with.

The relationship between a worker's causative theories and the subsequent interventions he makes is not, however, necessarily logical and consistent. For example, a neighbourhood worker may believe that the poor housing of the tenants was brought about by structurally determined inequities in the ownership, distribution and consumption of income, wealth and other resources. But his

97

or her mode of intervention with the tenants may be more or less the same as that of another worker who holds a different view about the causes of poor housing, who thinks that poor housing is an unfortunate dysfunction in a private and public housing market that on the whole operates to everyone's benefit. Both workers, with different theories of causation, might nevertheless intervene to organise the tenants into a group that could seek rehousing and the demolition of the slum.

There are, of course, other situations in which the neighbourhood worker's theories of causation will determine his interventions and distinguish them from those that another worker might make in the same situation. For example, local people might see their major problem as vandalism and delinquency in and around their tenement slum. One worker might say the 'cause' of the vandalism was associated with the poor housing conditions, while another worker would say it was caused by lack of recreational opportunities. The first worker would organise a tenants' housing action group, and the second worker might run a summer playscheme with a committee of interested parents. In this case, their interventions are different and follow from their individual causative theories. The first worker might also want to draw the group's attention to the relationship between their 'local' problem and those factors that he believes cause and shape the problem at city-wide, regional and national levels. Certainly, the nature of a worker's causative theories will determine the extent to which he or she is willing and able to set neighbourhood issues within a broader political and administrative context.

Recognition of Action About the Problem

The tasks of problem assessment might conclude with the worker setting down what has been discovered about people's readiness in the neighbourhood to take action in respect of the problem(s) they have mentioned. Besides *readiness* for action, the worker also needs to know what action various people think will be *effective*, and what they will *contribute* to that action by way of time, commitment, skills, resources, and so forth. There are thus three practice questions for the worker:

Are there any people who are ready to act?

If so, how do they want to act, and under what conditions will
they be prepared to act?
What are they willing to contribute to the action?

In order to ask and answer these questions, the worker will
need to differentiate between the various actors in the neighbourhood so far encountered. In particular, she will need to be clear
about:

the service agencies and other organisations who have shown an
interest in respect of the problem(s);
existing groups of residents who have expressed concern about
the problem(s);
any individuals who have said they would be willing to help, and
the conditions under which they will help.

The clarification of this information by the worker has two
purposes: first, it provides some preliminary data on residents that
will have to be considered in thinking about the feasibility of
particular goals and strategies; second, it helps to prepare for his
work in more systematically contacting groups and individuals
with a view to organising them for neighbourhood action of one
kind or another.

Setting Goals and Priorities

The next phase in working out what to do next is for the worker
to clarify her own goals and priorities, and those of the employing
agency. The necessity for considering goals and priorities is based
on the assumption that in most neighbourhoods the worker will
be faced with responding to more needs and demands than there is
the time, energy and resources to meet. Personal goal-setting as a
way of making a considered choice between the bits of work that
might be taken up does not imply pre-empting or encroaching
upon the decisions that local groups and people have to make
about *their* goals. Nor is personal goal-setting inimical to a
worker operating non-directively because this goal-setting pre-
cedes the worker's real engagement with local people and groups.
On the other hand, such personal goal-setting by the worker

may unwittingly *influence* those decisions that local people have to make. One cannot assume that any issue has as much chance as any other in being thrown up by the community. In practice, the knowledge and skills of its worker will have some influence, even without him wishing it, on the judgement of local people about what issues can viably be pursued.

Setting goals and priorities is largely concerned with:

choosing which of several 'competing' neighbourhoods or small geographical territories to focus on in respect of the problems and issues previously identified;

choosing which of a number of existing groups and organisations to work with, if any; and/or deciding what help to give to establishing new residents' organisations;

deciding whether or not to respond to the overtures and demands for help that will have by this stage come from agencies in the community;

deciding how to respond, if at all, to the demands made by one's own agency. Here the worker has to decide how much of the work will be focused on the neighbourhood, and how much on fostering change and development within his or her own agency; and finally,

deciding which of the identified problems/issues the worker will choose to pursue.

This last area of choice has two dimensions. First, the worker is likely to have identified a number of problems, most of which have salience for the people in the neighbourhood. She has to decide, in consultation with local people, groups and her own agency, which of these problem areas will be pursued; that is, she has to establish some priority among these problem areas, and some of the criteria by which this might be done has been suggested by Algie *et al.* (1977). In addition, the worker needs to take the following factors into account:

(1) The mandate and resources within the agency for pursuing the various problem areas. It may well be that a worker will have to give little or no priority to problems with which she and her agency have no mandate and authority to deal and in this kind of case the worker's task may be to 'refer' the problem to

workers in another agency who do have the appropriate mandate to intervene.

(2) Deciding on goals and priorities in the light of the worker's own experience, skills and interest. The worker must decide whether she has the right experience and skills to help people in respect of a particular problem, and whether or not she is *interested* in working with them on that particular problem.

(3) The worker's own values and preferences are an important element in establishing priorities, and choices made on the basis of the worker's values may conflict with choices suggested by agency-determined priorities, or by felt needs in the community. For example, a worker in a social services department may want, on the basis of personal values, to give priority to helping local people around the issue of bad housing, whilst her agency, and possibly some sections of the community, would attach more priority to establishing neighbourhood care schemes. Both worker and agency can justify their respective priorities in terms of agency mandate, resources and supporting data. The resolution of such a seeming impasse may be achieved only through a political and value-oriented dialogue, though at the end of the day the agency manager may use greater authority to ensure that the agency view of priorities prevails.

The second dimension of choice about problems is that of reducing banner statements of goals (there is a further discussion of goal setting in Chapter 7) to statements about sub-goals and the way in which they will be achieved. The sub-goals will represent an initial specification of the activities and strategies the worker will use in order to achieve major goals. For example, the worker might have chosen as a priority to 'run with' the issue of inadequate play facilities in the neighbourhood. Her banner goal statement might then read: 'to work on improving play facilities for X age group'. Some of the sub-goals that may be consequent on this major goal are shown in Figure 4.1.

The sub-goals are in effect instrumental goals through which the larger goal of improving play facilities may be achieved. The sub-goals specify the working targets for the worker, and as such they predict the range of roles and activities from which the worker can choose in order to achieve her particular targets. The worker

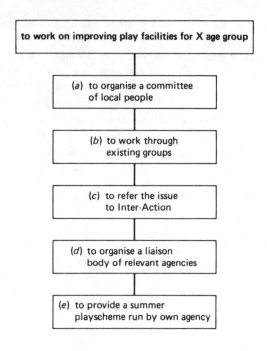

Figure 4.1 *An example of banner and sub-goals*

needs to be aware of the criteria to be used to decide upon which sub-goals to pursue. Such criteria include the following:

(1) Is the worker interested primarily in process or product results? That is, does she give priority to the learning goals that local people achieve through neighbourhood action, or is she more concerned to get tangible end-products into the neighbourhood? A worker interested in process goals will clearly choose sub-goals (a) and (b) in this particular case; whereas a worker who thinks it more important to get a play resource into the area may choose sub-goals (d) and (e) if she believes that working through agencies will produce the resources more quickly.

(2) How urgent is the need for an improvement in play facilities? If the worker is caught up in a crisis about vandalism and delinquency she may feel the pressure to provide an immediate playscheme, organised by herself and staffed with 'profes-

sional' workers; and only then feel able to move into organising local people around the issue of play.

(3) Which of the sub-goals is the worker best equipped to work on, in the way of time, energy, skills and experience?

(4) What constraints and opportunities attach to the worker's mandate, role and status, and to those of her agency, that seem to suggest that some sub-goals may be more feasible than others? It sometimes happens that a worker will be influenced in her choice of sub-goals by considering which are likely to be quickly achieved; this is often brought about by pressure on the worker from her agency to produce results.

Deciding on Role

Let us assume that the neighbourhood worker has to work at the task of getting people organised around the specific issues/problems that have been identified in the neighbourhood. Not only must the worker think about making contact with local people (see Chapter 5) but he must also consider the kind of role he is predisposed to play in his transactions with local people. We use the term 'predisposed' because we do not believe that workers should stick to a role or roles without regard to the situation in which they and the group find themselves. Sensitivity and flexibility are the key words to ensure that the neighbourhood worker adopts roles that will push forward, rather than hinder, the work of the neighbourhood group.

There is a proliferation of labels in community work literature that describe the roles open to the worker. 'Interpreter', 'communicator', 'enabler', 'guide', 'facilitator', 'encourager', 'catalyst', 'broker' and 'mediator' are labels that may be taken to suggest objective, neutral, democratic and even *laissez-faire* roles on the part of the worker; other words like 'stimulator', 'expeditor', 'organiser', 'negotiator', 'bargainer', 'advocate', 'expert' and 'activist' suggest more active or directive roles for the neighbourhood worker.

The proliferation of labels may confuse the practitioner who is intent on thoughtfully choosing the role(s) that seem most appropriate. He may be confused, first, because the proliferation of labels has not been fully matched by attempts to define the activities associated with them; second, the worker will find little consensus in the literature about either the extent of the range of roles open to him, the definitions of such roles, or their desirability or likely effectiveness; and, third, the elucidation of roles in the community work literature often conveys the impression that the worker's choice of role is an all-or-nothing commitment to one role, and a rejection of the others. We believe that the worker's choice of role should be a tactical or strategic decision, and that workers will move in and out of different roles according to particular circumstances. Within the context of directive and non-directive roles, Batten has suggested that there are a number of factors affecting this choice, including

> what the worker sees as people's major needs, and his thoughts about people who have these needs.
>
> the way in which he sees himself. 'Thus the more expert in diagnosing and meeting people's needs he feels himself to be, and the less he trusts the people he is working with to do this well enough for themselves, the more likely he is to choose a directive approach.'
>
> what he thinks will prove acceptable to the people he wants to work with. (1967).

Factors That Affect Role

In general, the choice of role might also be influenced by some or all of the following factors.

Type of Work   Rothman (1974a) has usefully suggested that the following roles are *primarily* associated wtih his three models of community organisation practice.

Locality Development:	enabler, catalyst, co-ordinator, teacher of problem-solving skills and ethical values
Social Planning:	fact-gatherer and analyst, programme implementer, facilitator
Social Action:	activist, advocate, agitator, broker, negotiator, partisan

Rothman is not suggesting that those roles are in practice or desirably confined to each mode of community work, or that the roles associated with, say, social planning are not appropriate or apparent in social action. Rather, he suggests that these roles are more salient than others in their respective modes of community work. It is clear that in so far as any piece of work will incorporate aspects of each of the three models then the worker will be called upon to play a large number of the salient roles.

Phases of Work We suggest that the phases or stages of neighbourhood work and point of development of the neighbourhood group's activities are among the key determinants of the roles to be played by the neighbourhood worker. Thomas, for instance, has suggested that the degree of directiveness or activism of the worker should vary according to the early, middle and closing phases of a group's life (1976). This same point can be made by looking at the worker's tasks in the different phases of intervention – it seems self-evident, for example, that the worker will need quite different roles in withdrawing from a group from those used in helping to recruit members to set it up.

The Goals of the Worker The nature of the relationship between a worker's goals and the roles that she adopts is something that has received little attention in the community work literature. Rothman's discussion of the relationship between goals and roles provides one of the few analyses (1969). Rothman indicates that there is no *necessary* relationship between non-directiveness and process goals, on the one hand, and, on the other, between directiveness and product goals. He also argues that role directiveness is not undemocratic:

> It is not the *act* of giving goal direction that may be questionable, but rather the *way* it is given. Within this logic, the practitioner . . . may validly suggest, advocate, and stimulate, as long as the approach is a factual and rational one, conveyed without entering into personalities and invective, without expressing primarily personal motives and desires, without bringing overbearing pressure, and, most important of all, as long as the final decision is left with the citizen group in which ultimate authority resides – and this lay prerogative is manifestly conveyed.

The value of stressing the *way* of giving goal direction is to confirm the point that the worker must give advice and suggest direction in a way which does not impair the freedom of the group to decline that advice.

What the Worker Likes Doing   We do not suggest that this is a major criterion to decide one's role predisposition because there are obvious risks to a group where a worker sticks stubbornly to roles that suit his likes and dislikes. Yet role effectiveness is in some way conditional upon the worker liking his role – and liking it from the point of view of its congruence with his values and feelings, as well as from satisfaction. What distinguishes the community worker is a disciplined use of self in his or her transactions with local groups – knowing when and how to contribute to the tasks and socio-emotional life of the neighbourhood group. This discipline may be contingent upon the worker being able, or having learnt, to *accept* the role and thus being able to function comfortably within it.

Agency Constraints and Opportunities   The neighbourhood worker's attempts to define roles must take into account, first, the expectations held of his role by his agency and colleagues, and, secondly, factors about an agency's values, structure and policies, that the worker can anticipate influencing his role options. For example, a neighbourhood worker from a local authority department may not be able to adopt a high-profile or 'front-line' role in a group's negotiations with that authority. As relevant as agency constraints is any expectation of role held within the local community.

Role Choice and Role Arenas

The notion of a continuum of directive/non-directive roles has been such a predominant influence in thinking about roles that it is very easy to fall into the trap of believing that a worker must be consistently directive or consistently non-directive. We suggest that the options about role that are open to the worker depend in large part on the nature of the *arena* in which she finds herself having to choose between roles. We suggest that there are three broad arenas, or situations, in which the worker will find herself and that of each of these has its own opportunities for the choice of role by the worker. The three arenas are:

relations with local people, either as individuals or in the group situation;

dealings between the group and other organisations in its environment;

transactions about the group within the worker's own agency, and between the worker and other agencies.

A worker can choose quite different roles according to the particular arena she finds herself in. It is possible for the worker to be a non-directive enabler in one situation, and a highly directive negotiator and advocate in another. We shall now explore these possibilities in more detail, though we are aware that these arenas are not so clear-cut and static in practice as we present them here.

Relations With Local People The directive/non-directive continuum seems appropriate only in considering role choice in relations with local people, and we suggest later that there are better ways of looking at role in respect of the two other arenas. Moreover, we believe that the degree of directiveness of the worker is a consideration that is largely relevant only to understanding *some* of the aspects of the worker's relations with local people; in particular the way in which the worker structures his or her contribution to group discussions and decision-making.

We see no value in being dogmatic or prescriptive about how directive or otherwise a worker should be. His or her choice in this matter must above all else be guided by a sense of pragmatism, with the choice being heavily influenced by what the worker sees as the needs of the group or of the individual in the particular situation. There is probably a strong case for neighbourhood workers to be *predisposed* to non-directiveness, but this does not mean that the worker should eschew more directive stances if these seem to be likely to be more helpful. The early stages of a group's life may call for a good deal of directive interventions by the worker, though in the last phases of a group the more appropriate stance might be that of non-directiveness.

Part of the difficulty that often faces students and workers about role choice is lack of clarity about what directiveness and

107

non-directiveness mean. They do suggest the bases of a continuum whose intermediate points remain unclear. In the next few pages, we propose to specify the different activities involved in directive and non-directive roles. First, let us start with directiveness, for degress of directiveness have already been suggested by Rothman (1969).

DIRECTIVENESS   Rothman suggests three points on the directive side of the continuum. These are:

Channelling   (strongly directive) 'The practitioner asserts a particular point of view with supporting arguments and documentation. He channels thinking directly toward a given goal.'

Funnelling   (considerably directive) 'This practitioner gives a range of possible choices and subtly funnels thinking in a given direction by asserting his preference for a particular goal and the rationale for that choice.'

Scanning   (mildly directive) 'This practitioner scans the range of possibilities related to solving a particular problem, presenting them impartially and on the basis of parity. He provides an orientation to goal selection, setting out the boundaries within which possible rational goal selection may take place.'

NON-DIRECTIVENESS   A great deal has been written about non-directiveness in community work and the classic texts are those of Batten (1967), the Biddles (1965, 1967) and Ross (1967). For Batten, the essence of non-directiveness 'is to create sufficiently favourable conditions for successful group action without in any way infringing group autonomy either by making decisions for the group or by doing for its members anything that they could reasonably be expected to do, or learn to do, for themselves'. In general the worker does this by:

trying to strengthen the incentives people have for acting together;
providing information about how other groups have organised;

helping people systematically to think through the problems they wish to deal with;

suggesting sources of any needed material help and technical advice;

helping to resolve any interpersonal difficulties between group members.

The Biddles develop their notion of non-directiveness by elaborating on the role of the community worker as *encourager*. It is extremely difficult to summarise the components of this role but it seems to comprise the activities of bringing people out of isolation; building optimism among local people; making internal conflict creative and 'making group life satisfying and productive'; and helping people to use experts without surrendering their autonomy to them. The personal qualities that an encourager should seek to exemplify are also discussed by the Biddles.

Murray Ross describes three roles for the community worker, those of *guide, enabler* and *expert*, and sees them as highly compatible and mutually supporting. He provides a clear exposition of the desirable behaviours and attitudes associated with each of these roles. In particular, his account of the role of enabler is one of the fullest expositions of non-directiveness in neighbourhood work. The work of the enabler involves:

focusing discontent on community conditions;
encouraging organisation;
nourishing good interpersonal relationships;
emphasising common objectives.

We need to know, however, *how* the enabler carries out these aspects of his work, and Ross's comments on this are:

As an enabler the worker seeks to facilitate the community process through listening and questioning; through identifying with, and in turn being the object of identification for, group leaders in the community; and by giving consistent encouragement and support to indigenous striving with common problems. He does not lead; he facilitates local efforts. He does not provide answers; he has questions which stimulate insight. He does not carry the burden of responsibility for organisation and action in the community; he provides encouragement and support for those who do.

The activity of *questioning* is central to the way in which the non-directive role is carried out, and to the way in which it is conceptualised by a number of the 'non-directive' writers. For Ross, questioning is a technique that the worker uses both to help the group in its 'here-and-now' discussions and 'to gain perspective, sense of movement, and fresh concern with long term objectives'. Batten stresses that the purpose of questioning is to help the group to *think*, 'by structuring, enlarging, and systematising the thinking process of the group'. The worker might intervene in a discussion, says Batten, in order to:

ensure that group members really are agreed about what they want to discuss;

ensure that they consider a range of possibilities and not just one;

keep discussion centred on one item at a time;

ensure that discussion in the group is based on facts and not on assumptions about facts;

ensure that the group is aware of factors it needs to take into account;

help to assess the progress that has been made and what still remains to be done.

Questioning as a technique, however, is not confined to neighbourhood workers who work in a traditional non-directive way. It is an important element of dialogical education and the 'conscientisation' process associated with Paulo Freire. It is, too, a technique used by workers who have traditionally been seen as outside the non-directive camp. For example, Saul Alinksy stresses the value of 'guided questioning' to the organiser:

The organiser's job is to inseminate an invitation for himself, to agitate, introduce ideas, get people pregnant with hope and a desire for change and to identify you as the person most qualified for this purpose. Here the tool of the organiser, in the agitation leading to the invitation as well as actual organisation and education of local leadership, is the use of the question, the Socratic method. (1971)

Having carried out this brief review of thinking on non-directiveness, we are now in a position to clarify further the role of the worker behaving in a non-directive fashion. We found it difficult to devise a continuum of non-directiveness, which in some ways is unfortunate because it would have fitted with Jack Rothman's continuum of directiveness. Clearly it is possible to think of non-directiveness as a continuum ranging from, say, scanning to *laissez-faire* but we have chosen to emphasise types of interventions in group processes and discussions that exemplify the non-directive role of the community worker. We suggest there are seven types of intervention to be associated with non-directiveness in the group situation. (In writing this, we have relied greatly on a mimeograph paper by Professor Frank Maple, 'The small group as a learning vehicle'.)

Galvanising The worker seeks to galvanise individuals or a group, stimulating their interest and their morale and mobilising them either to form a group, or if in one, to stick to working out its goals and tasks. The worker does this by the following means:

Supportive behaviour and interventions. Rothman says of this that the practitioner 'lends support to various opinions or sentiments that arise in the community concerning the problem. He stimulates community morale and activity through his presence, his encouragement, his indications that he is aware of the community's problems and sympathises with its attempts to cope with them.'

Strengthening incentives for people to take action. Batten suggests that the worker does this by helping people to restate their needs in terms of specific wants and goals to be achieved.

Inspiring people with a vision of what can be achieved in the neighbourhood by local people coming together. Both Alinsky and Warren Haggstrom have written about the contribution of the worker's vision, and Haggstrom has written of its mobilising effects as follows:

An organiser must not only perceive how people are, but it is also essential that he be *unrealistic* in that he perceives people as they can be. Noting what is possible, the organiser projects this possibility and moves people to accept it and to seek to realise it. The organiser helps people to develop and live in an alternative reality in which their image of themselves and their abilities is enhanced . . . People are moved to accept the new world of which they catch a glimpse because it appears to be attainable in practice and intrinsically superior to the world in which they have been living. (1970)

There is further discussion of galvanising in the next chapter.

Focusing This activity by the neighbourhood worker helps to keep the group focused on the task at hand. The focuser follows three rules.

He does not get into competition with other group members.
He shows support (creates a positive environment) for any idea that a member voices.
He should keep interest at a high level, mainly through demanding and asking difficult questions.

Clarifying The worker intervenes here in order to ensure that:

people are clear about the purposes of the discussion, and the task the group is working on;
the comments and questions of individual members are unambiguous and understood by all;
real consensus has been reached before the group moves on to discuss another agenda item.

Summarising The purpose of summarising is to help the group to take stock of discussions, and to assess how much progress has been made towards completing its task. The worker intervenes to condense the group's discussion to a few sentences. Summarising may be seen as an intervention that helps the movement of the group through the various stages of its discussion.

Gate-keeping This type of intervention by the worker is designed to ensure that each of the members in the group has an opportunity to contribute to discussion. This means encouraging participants who say little and helping to limit the contributions of others who are more dominant in the discussion.

Mediating This intervention seeks to resolve interpersonal disagreements between members that the worker believes are a threat to the group attaining its discussion objectives. Too much energy can be dissipated in a group on negative relationships between members.

Informing The worker facilitates discussion in the group by acting as an informant about:

resources and advice that the group might need to make decisions;
facts that the group needs in its discussions;
the experiences of other groups in reaching decisions about similar kinds of issues.

It must be emphasised that these above seven functions in the group process are not the prerogative of the neighbourhood worker. They are, of course, functions that are, and ought to be, 'shared' among all the members of a group. We suggest only that it is through taking up one or several of these functions during a group meeting that the worker is able to contribute non-directively to the discussion.

Dealings Between the Group and Other Organisations The labels that conventionally define the role of the neighbourhood worker at the interface of the group and more formal and established organisations include broker, mediator, advocate, negotiator and bargainer. They immediately convey the sense of greater worker autonomy and activism, though it is not the case that the nature of these interface roles determines or predicts the roles the worker plays *within* the group situation. The worker may, of course, take or be given more of a leadership role at the interface but remain inside the boundary of non-directiveness with his relations with local people.

Neighbourhood groups have to deal with a number of other systems, including local authority departments, branch offices of central government departments and other groups in the community. Such transactions might include meetings, deputations, petitions, demonstrations, holding a press conference, negotiating for money and other resources, lobbying, and so on. For each of these transactions the group and the worker must give thought to what role the worker will play. If there is to be a meeting with elected members about a particular issue, is the worker to come along? If he or she is, will she play the role of observer/recorder, or will she be given the mandate to intervene as she thinks necessary?

The critical first step for group and worker to take in respect of the worker's role is to realise and accept that this question of role needs to be thought about, discussed and decided upon. It is all too easy in the rush and turmoil of preparing for a meeting to neglect to discuss the worker's contribution, if any (indeed, many groups are less than effective in such meetings largely because they have failed to discuss *member* roles adequately). It is especially important to be clear in what capacity the worker will be attending – as a representative of the group or of her agency?

The notion of representation is a helpful one in understanding the worker's role in dealings with other organisations. In most cases, the worker will be attending as a representative of the group, and indeed the members of a committee who go to a meeting are also representatives of that committee and of its wider constituency in the neighbourhood. Rice (1965) has differentiated between three kinds of representation – observer, delegate, plenipotentiary – and these are helpful in understanding the neighbourhood worker's degree of activism and autonomy in negotiations between the group and other systems.

OBSERVER/RECORDER   Here the worker's job consists solely of observing and taking notes of what occurs. The neighbourhood group has not given her the mandate to express any views or intervene in the discussion. Her presence may also be a support to the group and an unsettling factor to 'the other side'.

DELEGATE   In this role, the worker is given a set piece to say, either at some agreed point in the transactions or at her discretion. For example, the worker might be asked by the group to present the statistical side of the case it is making to decision-makers, and it is understood that the worker will confine her contribution to giving this information. She has no authority to go outside this brief.

PLENIPOTENTIARY   In this role, it is only the predetermined goals and policies of the group that provide limits on the negotiating power of the worker in transactions with other systems. She, and perhaps the group members, are given a flexible and open-ended mandate to contribute to the discussion as she thinks fit.

The final point to make about these three kinds of representation is that they can, of course, be used to understand the kind of mandate a committee or constituency will give to a delegation. Very often in community work, delegations get into trouble with their committee, and the committee with its constituency, because the delegation was not given, and did not itself establish, whether it had observer, delegate or plenipotentiary powers in its negotiations with outside systems. The consequence of this absence of clarity is that delegations often commit their committees to courses of action when they were not empowered to do so.

Transactions About the Group in the Worker's Agency Neighbourhood workers are rightly wary of being put in the position of spokesman or go-between for community groups. Yet in their own agency they may be asked to comment on some matter that concerns the community group they work with, or other agencies may contact them to give or to ask for information about the group. In most of these situations the worker will attempt to get the inquirers to make direct contact with the local group, offering perhaps the telephone number or address of the relevant officer. Within the group, the worker may be also seen as spokesman or representative of his agency or even of the local authority, and again he may see his role as putting local people in direct contact with those agency staff who can best help them with the particular inquiry.

This re-routing function may constitute, together with the passing on of information and intelligence, the lowest level of activism for the worker in his agency setting. There is, however, need to consider that opportunities for a more high-profile role will often arise. For example, a practitioner working with homeless families may find herself in situations where she can promote their general and specific interests through her contributions to agency discussions. She may be able to seize opportunities to promote an organisational or policy change that is in their interests. A person working on play issues with a group may suddenly become aware of unallocated resources available in the department. Clearly situations will occur in which the neighbourhood worker will be pressured to make a decision that concerns the work of a group without being able fully to refer the matter back to the group. These may be the types of situation the worker would much prefer to avoid but there will be times when this is not possible. What is he to do? Does he make a bid to secure the unallocated resources for the group or does he sit quietly, because he has not been able to consult the group, and let the resources be put to some other use in the agency or community?

There is no easy answer or prescription for dealing with such situations but the fact that they occur ought to be discussed between the worker and the group. It might then be possible for each to establish guidelines to help the worker to handle better his linkage role between agency and group. The making explicit of the worker's status as an agency employee, and how he is to manage his roles of employee and group worker, serves another important purpose. It should help both the worker and the group not to be seduced into seeing the worker as just another group member, and to recognise the potential stress for the worker in feeling accountable both to his agency and to the community group. There is little value in the worker and the group 'pretending' that the worker is a full member because events will occur when the worker will have to say 'I'm sorry, but I can't do this with you' and this sudden revelation may undermine the confidence of the group.

We have, then, discussed three different arenas which suggest different role possibilities for the community worker. The purpose of this extended discussion of role has been to free our discussion (and the worker's choice) of role from the constraints that are imposed both by traditional role labels and by the blanket application of the directive/non-directive polarity. We now move to discuss the fourth element of working out what to do next.

Specification of the Next Moves

The neighbourhood worker must now use previously developed statements about problems, goals, skills and roles to decide how to move into, and carry out, the next task of making contact with local people in order to form an organisation around the salient issue or problem. In other words, the worker needs to think about and specify next steps as they seem predicted by earlier assessments and decisions.

Let us assume a worker has, when sorting our her goals and priorities, decided to organise local residents around the issue of play. She has given some preliminary thought to her own skills and interests in this task, and anticipated the variety of roles she may be called upon to play. She now has to decide and estimate *method, time* and *resources*. She has to ask herself: *how* will I organise local people? and what time and resources will be demanded from me and other people? In addition, the worker might also anticipate any difficulties and resistances she might encounter, and how she will overcome or circumvent them. Her planning tasks may be portrayed as follows:

Major Objectives: To organise a group of local people around the issue of play.

Method: Here the worker must consider the various alternatives open to her of identifying, meeting and encouraging people to form a group. She needs to evaluate the likely costs and benefits of each approach and technique, and specify what they will demand of her skills, time and other resources. Different methods of forming a group are discussed in the next two chapters.

Resistance: What factors can the worker anticipate will frustrate, hinder or delay her intervention? There seem to be two categories: those within the community (e.g. apathy, suspicion, fragmentation) and those in her agency and other institutions (lack of mandate, support, understanding, facilities). Conversely, the worker should anticipate those factors that will help and facilitate her intervention.

Circumvention: The worker then thinks about how these resistances can be circumvented and blockages removed, and she may have to modify her original plan if she anticipates being able to do little about the predicted resistance.

117

Reporting and
Assessment:
The worker must also plan how she will record her intervention to organise a group, and the purposes for which she will record. One important purpose of record-keeping is to facilitate the monitoring and assessment of the intervention. The worker must be prepared to alter her problem choice, major objective and method if further contact with local people provides evidence to question her earlier assessments and decisions.

Summary

This chapter has stressed the importance of planning as an integral element of the neighbourhood work process. We are aware, however, of the possible dangers to action, in particular that preparation and planning can be used to put off and delay intervention. We have indicated already that the early stages are probably the most stressful for the neighbourhood worker and some workers may be tempted to prolong planning in order to stay off the streets, as it were. Clearly, workers and agency supervisors need to be alert to this possibility.

On the other hand, we suggest that planning and reflection of the kind we have described in this chapter may be a way of mitigating the stress of the first stages of neighbourhood work by guiding the worker through the various activities and stages of his or her intervention. However, no amount of planning and preparation will enable the worker to predict all the variables in a turbulent community environment that will shape and distort his work, and so his guided intervention needs to remain responsive to the influences and events he encounters as he goes about making contact with local residents.

CHAPTER 5

Making Contacts and Bringing People Together

This chapter is about the neighbourhood worker making contact with local people. The task of the worker is to meet residents in order to identify their interest in collective action and the possible contributions they might make, and to bring them together with other individuals. The purpose is to help people form a group, and Chapter 6 deals with the transformation of a group into an organisation that represents a constituency on whose behalf the organisation will act.

Methods and skills in making contact with people are essential through the whole neighbourhood work process, so we must stress that *many of the ideas and techniques discussed as part of this phase are relevant within all the other phases of the process.* The particular phase of making contacts in order to get people into a group is, however, especially crucial for the worker. Failure here means that the process of getting people organised can hardly start. The ways in which the worker initially relates to residents and helps them explore the possibilities of collective action are likely to affect their later development and goals as a community organisation.

Encouraging people to form a group or network demands a complexity of skills on the part of the worker. It is, too, a phase of neighbourhood work in which the worker will again feel isolated and vulnerable, moving between states of elation and depression as residents respond positively or negatively to her encouragement. The worker is at risk of assimilating the doubts and despair that are voiced by both local people and agency personnel, and she will often be harassed by an internal need and an external expectation (again from local residents and agency workers) to achieve something – preferably soon and tangible.

There are other sources of stress in this phase of the work. The worker may have strong doubts about her legitimacy and credibility for intervening in a community. She may also feel uncertain about the best ways of making contact with people. She wants answers for the following sorts of questions. How do I approach people? Do I knock on a door or stop someone in the street? How will I introduce myself? Will they understand what I say? Will they talk to me? What business have I to confront local people about problems in their area? While it may be all right for male workers to knock on doors and approach strangers, what do they think when they see me, a woman, engaged in these activities? The community can so easily become for the worker an undifferentiated and unreceptive entity, some of whose members may be openly hostile and rejecting of the worker's efforts to make contacts.

Many of these doubts and anxieties are stimulated by the fact that most workers *are* outsiders and strangers. It may be that neighbourhood workers do not always appreciate the extent to which they are strangers to the community they wish to serve. Many workers may have a strong sense of identification with the needs and problems of the inhabitants of an area but may be unaware that their feelings of attachment are not reciprocated; workers may not realise that their identification and commitment do little to mediate between their status as an outsider and the continuing problems (and distrust of professionals) of the neighbourhood.

It is natural for workers to assume that there is in the community an understanding and appreciation of their work that will easily overcome suspicion about their motivation to help. The very closeness of relationships that often develops between a worker and a neighbourhood group can lead even the most experienced worker to fudge over the marginality of his position with local people, which exists even when he is well known to the members of a group, and even after he has been tested and 'accepted'. How much more marginal is the position of the worker at the time he attempts to initiate contact with local residents!

Apprehension – even fear – of what will be encountered will clearly vary with the type of person the worker is, and the kind of community in which he or she seeks to intervene. But being scared to one degree or another may be an inevitable part of this phase of the work. One worker has graphically described some of the sources of this fear:

Recognize the fact that the organizer who comes into the community for the first time is internally in a precarious position. He is afraid – or at least he should be if he has any brains that he doesn't want beaten out.

He is afraid because he doesn't know the people, and we are all vaguely afraid of people we don't know. If he is white and he is going to work in a black community, he is doubly afraid. If he is a middle-class black, he is afraid too, for similar but not quite identical reasons.

He is afraid because he is the bearer of a new idea. Mankind does not cotton on to new ideas in general, but especially not to the new ideas that organizers bring. This is so because they may mean trouble and because the organizer's presence says, in effect, 'You are so dumb that you need me to think your way out of this mess you are in.' Don't kid yourself about this. Nothing absolves the organizer of this sin.

The organizer is also afraid because a failure is a crushing blow to his ego or his self-respect. Even a bad organizer puts a tremendous part of himself on the line when he goes into a community. In his own eyes, he is being tried as a person, as a huge test of his own worth. To fail is to be adjudged as a capon, a sexless, impotent thing by one's self, or so I always found it.

These fears work on most organizers to make them very susceptible to thinking the people they meet in the community who are sympathetic are the people to listen to and work with. I can't count the number of times I have wandered into communities to find the people who were supposed to be building a mass organization mucking around with pious, middle-class clergymen or teenagers (Von Hoffman, 1972).

Von Hoffman's last comment is suggestive of yet another source of doubt and anxiety for the worker in this stage of the process. The task of identifying 'leaders' or, more generally, of recruiting people to form a group may appear to the worker to depend too much on chance and opportunism rather than on judgement and skills. Success in making the right contacts may seem determined by many factors outside a worker's control. If the worker happens to be in the right pub at the right time on the right day she may meet the indigenous community leader most able to take forward the organisation of a group; if she is not there, the group may go forward in a completely different way, with different personalities and interests.

But how does she *know* when she meets the people most likely to help to get a group going? What criteria does she use to assess people's likely contribution to collective action? And is it her business, anyway, to select out people – is community work not supposed to be about enabling the least motivated and able to take part in community affairs? Von Hoffman again indicates some of the difficulties for the worker:

> ... plucking out 'natural leaders' by dint of casual observation and conversation is very chancy. I recall having picked a number of these on-first-sight gems and I also recall spending months kicking myself for having done so.
>
> The guy who is indeed the most natural small-group leader may turn out to be the guy who gets hopelessly and permanently confused by committees or simply by having to keep in mind that now instead of dealing with ten old faithfuls in the block club he's got to worry about what 400 people think. The guy with the big line about how 'it's about time the black man showed those m-fs' can turn out to be one great big chicken, or what can be worse yet, a lazy bum who only comes to meetings to make long theatrical monologues.
>
> The leaders in the third month of an organization's life are seldom the leaders in the third year; a few leaders, ourselves included, are really all-purpose; and the best organizations create a 'collective leadership'.
>
> The first leadership is usually the closest leadership at hand. It is usually selected in the enthusiasm of the first campaign, because it is available. You don't have a choice and you have to go with what you've got ...

But you will notice too that the reasons for your picking the first leaders (and you know it's you who picks them) say nothing about how they will wear out over a period of time. That respectable clergyman can turn out to be a timid jerk; the lady who was so good at sounding off in front of the judge may be good for nothing else; and that big freedom fighter can look like a vain egomaniac living off the reputation of a deed done many years ago.

The lesson I draw from this is that at the beginning keep the organization very loose, and spread the responsibilities and the conspicuous places around. This permits you, and the new membership that you are supposed to be recruiting, to judge the talent, and it keeps things sufficiently porous so that new talent isn't blocked off. Nothing is more absurd than an organization that's six months old, without a dime in the treasury and a membership that can fit in a Volkswagen, having a cemented-in, piggy leadership. Vested interests are only tolerable when they are protecting something of value, not fancy organizational charts, letterheads, and research programs.

Don't laugh. This kind of thing is a clear and present danger. (1972)

We continue the discussion about the identification of leadership in the next chapter.

The need to identify and commit oneself to *people* is not the only source of concern for the worker who has, too, to help residents to identify an interest in a *problem* or *issue*. The worker will wonder what criteria to use to decide on what is a 'good' problem to work with.

How the worker makes judgements about people and problems highlights a major 'policy' decision that workers will often face in these opening moves of neighbourhood work. There seem to be two different situations that may confront a worker as the process of group formation begins.

The first is where the worker's goal is to enable a specific group of people to organise for community action – the worker has a sense of *whom to organise* (e.g. the tenants of a housing estate) and the tasks are to determine the pragmatic means by which to do so, including the identification of the issues around which people are likely to organise.

In the second situation, the worker's goal is to generate some group action in respect of a specific need – the worker wants to do something about a *particular problem* (e.g. poor housing, lack of recreational facilities) and the major tasks are the identification and recruitment of appropriate individuals, groups and organisations. In both situations, the worker has to build up contacts with local residents, not just as individuals, but perhaps as members of neighbourhood groups that are already in existence.

The issue of whether to work through an existing organisation or to by-pass it and help create another is often a testing one for the neighbourhood worker. The issue is crucial in a 'closed' community like a housing estate where there would seem to be little 'room' for a new organisation, and where the attempt to generate something new may lead to animosities not only between the worker and the existing group but between neighbours and friends.

On the other hand, a new group may be preferable if existing groups are unrepresentative of the goals and ambitions of the community, or where it pursues interests that do not address the concerns of most people. A typical example is a tenants' association that refuses to enlarge on its role of running a bar and other social facilities and will not take up housing and other issues of concern to the tenants. Some existing groups may also be prejudiced against the interests of minority sections of the community, and these can be protected only by forming alternative organisations. The difficulty for the neighbourhood worker is that he may be acutely aware of the deficiencies of existing groups, but be just as aware of the pitfalls in trying to circumvent them.

Making Contact: But for What Reasons?

We are primarily concerned in this chapter with making contact on a person-by-person basis. We see other forms of contact-making, such as by letter or telephone, as relevant only when they precede and thus facilitate personal contact and understanding. What we have to consider is how the worker sets about *engaging* with potential members of a community group, or with actual members of an existing group(s).

At one level it seems very self-evident why the neighbourhood worker has to make contact with local people: he cannot carry out his work if he does not make relationships with them. But there are more specific purposes behind this phase of making contact.

(1) *Giving people the opportunity to get to know the worker and to form some initial assessment of the worker as a person.* The associate director of a Community Action Programme vividly describes the importance of this.

> Now it's like this. When you're dealing with people downtown or in some big organization, it's important to tell them who you are – your title, what you expect to accomplish, and the like. You play it like an organizational 'rep'. But when you're in the neighbourhood, people don't want to know your title. They want to know *you*. Can they trust you? Are you afraid of getting your hands dirty? Are you going to play square or just promise the world?
>
> I talk plain, straight from the shoulder over a cup of coffee or a beer. I never make promises. I always stress that 'we' (them and us) have a problem. If I told them all the resources I was going to bring in or used a bunch of bureaucratic words, they would throw me out on my ear. If a guy uses big fancy words and I don't know what he's talking about, I'd walk out, or toss him out.
>
> Once they get to know you, then you talk about your organization – but only about how it might help them deal with the problems and the gripes they've already shared with you.
> (Quoted in Ecklein and Lauffer, 1972)

Local people need to find out how reliable the worker is or is likely to be; where her loyalties lie; how she sees the neighbourhood and understands the people who live in it and the problems they face; how she responds to different kinds of people and situations in the neighbourhood; and various aspects of the worker's personality, beliefs and values that are in themselves important to local people or provide clues as to how useful the worker is going to be to any group that might form.

(2) *Presenting information about the worker's role, organisation and what he or she has to offer.* Among the factors that some people will take into account in weighing up the costs and benefits of getting involved in community action will be their understanding of the part and role the worker will play. They may also be

interested in the resources that can be opened up through the worker's own role and skills, and of any resources he or she may be able to bring. The worker must be specific and frank enough for people to be able to assess his potential contribution; yet not so intrusive that it seems to be more salient than the roles, skills and resources of the community, and not so dominating that it fosters a sense of dependence.

The difficulties facing a worker coming from a community work project are that people will find it hard to understand the auspices and function of the project; whereas for workers employed in an established agency like the social services or chief executive's office the problem is almost a contrary one: people will often have quite well-formed views on the function of the agency; the worker may have difficulty in describing his role in ways that distinguish his particular contribution from those of other personnel from the agency already known to residents.

The effective presentation by the worker of self, role and organisation (as well, perhaps, as his previous experience) will contribute to establishing his identity – 'getting his licence to operate'. The concreteness and credibility of his identity will depend on conclusions about him that people derive not only from the information he presents about his person, role and sponsor, but also on the *way* he presents it. Not only will people take clues about him from such things as his dress, language and life-style but the answers that the worker gives to people's questions such as 'What's in it for him?', 'What's he really after?', 'Who is paying him to do this and why?' must be acceptable within the experience of the community.

(3) *Motivating, or galvanising, residents to consider the possibilities of community action.* Galvanisation comprises a number of activities including developing people's awareness about issues in an area, exploring the costs and benefits of collective action, alerting people to the range of skills and resources they have or are available to them, and motivating them by establishing a sense of their general competence and confidence. It is not enough for people to become persuaded only of the worker's skills and competence – they must also be given faith in their own abilities and strength.

Galvanisation involves both *reflection* and *vision*. Reflection, meaning an internal process of conceptualisation and reasoning, is

126

a means through which people and groups overcome what Rowbotham has called a 'paralysis of consciousness' (1974) and become able to understand, conceptualise and articulate what goes on around them and impinges on their social, economic and political lives. Reflection of this kind may produce an understanding of how to intervene to affect these forces, and to predict, control and overcome them.

Techniques to facilitate reflection have been developed and used by community workers. Alinsky, in particular, is well known for his repertoire of interventions designed to stimulate people into a thinking awareness of their situation. Much of his writing emphasises the importance of reflection and he argues, for instance, that 'the function of the organiser is to raise questions that agitate, that break through the accepted pattern . . . [to raise] . . . the internal questions within individuals that are so essential for the revolution which is external to the individual' (1971).

British workers have also described their techniques for promoting reflection. One of these techniques that is being used more and more as an educational, consciousness-raising tool in community work is video. Video, and an analysis of its strengths and limitations in community work, are discussed later in the chapter.

Reflection enables people to understand the situations that limit them and to attempt to overcome them. *Vision* follows on from reflection – increased consciousness of me-in-this-situation can lead to a vision of me-in-another-situation in the future.

Effective action is contingent upon local people being able to conceive of themselves as 'new' people – a conception of themselves working at tasks, taking on roles and exercising skills and knowledge in ways previously unimaginable to them. The neighbourhood worker's task is to help people to articulate a desired future state of affairs (such as better housing, a new playground), and then to work with them to realise it. The challenge facing the worker, however, is that before people become organised, group members are often not visionary. They may perceive something is wrong, but often they do not know what they want to do by way of improving the situation, or how to go about it. The worker's task, then, is to develop in people a capacity for visionary thought, to help them cross what Freire

127

has called 'the frontier which separates being from being more'.

The neighbourhood worker will often be purposively catalytic in galvanising group members to cross the frontier between 'being and being more'. The worker can do this by using his own vision of a better world to inspire group members, and a consumer's view of the galvanising effect of the worker's vision is given in an account of a worker's intervention in the Crimea Road part of 'Waychester':

> after the initial success of the public meeting, constant drives for new membership were needed to involve more people as interest flagged amongst the original contacts. There was a complete turnover in the first couple of months and only one of the original contacts formed part of the group that finally got the playgroup off the ground. Everything seemed to depend on the community worker's energy and ability to motivate people: 'James was charismatic – his enthusiasm would fill *us* with enthusiasm – we'd feel "This is possible. We can actually do this!" He was always bounding off into new areas.' (Taylor *et al.*, 1976)

Moving people to accept a 'new world' requires at least three things of the neighbourhood worker. First, that he works with residents to develop an appropriate organisation and decision-making processes; second, that he works with them to transform visionary statements into operational goals; and third, that he helps people to see leadership as located not just in himself but in themselves and other members of the group. The skills that are required of the neighbourhood worker are not just those of knowing when and how to inspire people by sharing his vision and enthusiasm about their capabilities; but also those of doing so without appearing unrealistic or naive, and without seeming to impose his preconceptions about what the specific goals and strategies of the community effort might be.

(4) *Finally, increasing his knowledge of people and their lives in the neighbourhood*. This has two essential aspects. First, that of consolidating information about residents that was gathered in the earlier data-gathering phase of the intervention. Second, encouraging people to form a group around the issue or grievance in question; and, in particular, looking for residents who might occupy key leadership positions in any group that is formed. This

aspect of contact-making has been called *searching for a constituency*.

In summary we suggest that the important purposes to be achieved in the phase of making contact are to give and receive information about oneself and residents; to establish one's identity and identification with local people; to create rapport and the basis of trust and understanding; to affect attitudes and motivations about individuals' competence and the potential of collective action; to identify points of contact and intervention of mutual interest, and thus to clarify areas of 'goal convergence' between oneself and residents; and to begin to describe a provisional agenda for the involvement of worker and residents in the formation of a group. All of these indicate the substantive difference between making contact at this stage in the neighbourhood work process and the more limited engagement with the community described in Chapter 2.

The Process of Making Contact

It should be very evident by now that making contact is about verbal and non-verbal communication – it is a process of discussion, dialogue, questioning, listening and understanding. Contacts with local people may be differently perceived as 'conversations' or 'interviews'. If a worker sees them as conversations they may be viewed more as a pleasurable activity, an art-form, in which the social and work aspects of the contact are hard to separate out. For example, the Biddles describe contact-making in terms of informal conversations:

> Such an informal exchange with individuals occurs most often in homes or in other places where people feel 'at home'. Motivations that may have been mistakenly attributed to him can be changed gradually by simple friendliness as the encourager (the community worker) listens to other people's conversations and shares in their worries. There is an art of creative listening and sympathising. There is also an art of raising questions that invite the other person to talk about those things that are dear to him. Especially important is the skill that enables the other person to make articulate the concerns, fears, and frustrations that make life difficult for him. (1968)

The tendency to view contacts as conversations rather than interviews will be strengthened by feelings that the notion of an 'interview' jars with the worker's perception of the participatory, even peer, basis of contacts with local people. Another kind of perspective on contacts as conversation is that conversations are an integral part of working-class political education. For example, a community worker in North Shields emphasises how the conversation that occurs in shops, pubs and clubs is part of the everyday political exchanges that take place between residents (Foster, 1975).

The view of contacts that is perhaps at the opposite end of the continuum will see them more as interviews than conversations. Seeing contacts as interviews alerts one to the need to plan and prepare for them, to see them primarily as an instrumental and not a social activity, and to associate them with specific techniques and skills for carrying them out effectively. This approach to contacts is put most strongly by Brager and Specht, and is also reflected in the laboratory programmes for students that have been established on some community work courses. Referring their readers to the 'considerable material on the uses and techniques of interviewing in the literature', Brager and Specht write:

> interviewing may be distinguished from conversation on three important grounds: (1) it is *goal-oriented*, that is, the worker has a purpose, something that he wishes to come out of the contact; (2) it is *self-conscious* in that he is thoughtful about the interaction and his own role in it; and (3) it is *focused*, that is, the worker selects his questions and responses in the context of his purposes. Although the above may sound imposing and overformal, experienced interviewers can be friendly and warm, if required, without violating these strictures. (1973)

The polarisation of views about whether contacts are conversations or interviews is helpful only if it enables us to recognise that contacts should best be seen as embodying elements of both conversation and interview. Contact-making in neighbourhood work ought to be both friendly, sociable, caring and receptive, as well as focused, purposeful and goal-directed. A balance has to be achieved between these elements; there is no point in the worker who is looking for information so structuring the contact that the other person becomes hostile and the worker fails to establish rapport and the basis for continuing work. On the other hand, there is limited value in a contact where the worker and other person get on famously together but the worker fails to acquire the information that he wants.

We suggest that the process of contact-making may helpfully be seen as comprising three stages.

Preparing for the Contact

This consists of the following planning or preparation activities.

(1) *Selecting people to talk to, and the sequence in which to do so.* Time can be wasted in talking with the 'wrong' people (wrong, perhaps, because with a bit of foresight you might have seen they could not add to what other people have already told you); goodwill can be endangered by omitting to see people who think you *ought* to see them; and feathers and thus co-operativeness can be ruffled if there's a pecking order in the neighbourhood and you contacted people 'out of order'.

(2) *Selecting a setting in which to meet people.* Two considerations should guide the selection of the setting. First, the purpose of the meeting: if the worker wants an extended and perhaps confidential discussion a noisy crowded pub with its distractions for the other person of friends and neighbours may not be the best place; such a setting would be appropriate, however, if the worker wanted to use the meeting to get to know other people. Second, local attitudes to where meetings should be held: a particular pub or cafe may not be a 'respectable' place to meet, or residents may feel reluctant to invite a relative stranger into their homes.

(3) *Deciding what you want to get out of the contact.* Is it information about some community issue or event, or the presentation of oneself as an interested and resourceful worker, or change in the other person's attitudes and behaviour, or introductions to other people in the area? Of course, the worker may have a number of goals for the contact, and so she will have to decide which of them has priority.

(4) *Deciding on the means through which you will achieve the goals of the meeting.* Are there points of influence you can bring to bear to get the information or interest that you seek? What questions do you have to ask to get the information you seek from

the other person? What will you be prepared to give to the other person in return for the help he can give?

(5) *Deciding on how you will present yourself, your agency and your interests.* This involves trying to anticipate and thus minimise any negative forces that may be at work in the meeting that derive from factors such as the personal attributes of the worker (e.g. age, sex, race), the status of the agency, and the other person's previous experience of neighbourhood work. The worker must also anticipate and make the most of positive forces in the situation. In brief, the worker must think how she will manage her image in her contact with different local people, though this does not entail giving up her integrity or behaving unlike her real self. Von Hoffman provides some interesting comments on image management and the way in which the organiser comes across to local people.

> People may admire youth, they may praise, they may believe that youth is showing the way in which age should follow, but they are very, very reluctant to trust youth with anything of immediate value . . .
> Impressions do count. I'll mention clothes. It is one thing to wear overalls in Mississippi where many of the people actually do wear them – it is another to wear them as an occasional stunt in a big Northern city. To indulge in peculiarities of dress and speech simply makes you look like faddists . . .
> Drop as much of your excess ideological baggage as you can . . . don't act like cultists. If you are a vegetarian, keep it to yourself, hide it, because there are a certain number of butchers in the community, and you want them in the organisation too. (1972)

A further aspect of anticipating the contact is that of rehearsing it, though without detracting from the spontaneity that must be present. Contact may be rehearsed through discussing it with a colleague or through role play. Jacobs has written of his experience that the warmth of the welcome he received from one couple indicated 'all nervousness and prior rehearsing on how best to introduce the project to have been unnecessary' (1976). Perhaps the contact developed so well precisely because the worker had spent some time in preparing for it.

The Contact

The task of the neighbourhood worker in any contact with local people is both to establish rapport and to achieve the outcomes for the contact that she has previously specified. Establishing rapport may itself be the goal and it is doubtful that other goals (such as getting information about a community issue) would be achieved without some rapport between the worker and the other person. Brager and Specht have defined some of the elements of establishing rapport in a community work setting. They are that the worker is able to be accepting of others; to empathise; to tolerate feedback (about for instance, himself, his intentions or his agency); to accept and even encourage socially or worker unacceptable views; and to be able to 'speak the language' of the people though aware of the dangers of being patronising and ingratiating. (Alinsky's phrase of 'speaking within the experience of the community' is a better one.)

It may be difficult to think about rapport in a purposeful way. To do so seems to conflict with views that rapport is essentially to do with the 'chemistry' between two people, something that is outside the influence of the people concerned. It may seem inappropriate to think that there may be things one can do – guidelines to follow – that maximise positive and minimise negative rapport. Thinking in these terms might also be distasteful to workers who detect undertones of manipulation. For these and other reasons more may be learnt about establishing rapport from the field of participant observation, and Bogdan and Taylor (1975) have written about rapport in a way which neighbourhood workers will find helpful.

Bearing in mind the twin tasks of establishing rapport and conducting the contact in such a way that the worker achieves the outcomes he or she has specified, we suggest that the actual contact with the other person may be seen as comprising the following activities.

(1) *Crossing the boundary.* This may be that of a person's flat, or the door in the bar of a public house. Different kinds of boundary pose different kinds of problems and challenges to different workers. The main task in boundary crossing is to take stock of the immediate environment in which the contact is to happen. The worker must decide on how to cope with factors in the environment that, for instance, may detract from the value of

the contact; for example, there may be a noisy television in the room or a group of children at play, both of which might distract the attention of the worker and other person; the seating arrangements may be inappropriate; or there may be friends and neighbours present and the worker may not be sure how they will affect the progress of the contact.

(2) *Introducing oneself.* Neighbourhood workers may be uncertain about how detailed, frank and specific their introductions should be; some will see an emphasis on introductions as working against establishing rapport and a sense of ease; whilst others would feel that introductions are important so that the other person is aware of the nature and implications of the contact. The worker must introduce himself and his agency and give the other person an idea of what his purposes are, and why the other person has been chosen to be interviewed. It might help, too, to suggest the possible areas for discussion in the interview. Our experience from our skills workshops is that workers tend to give too little information or too much. In giving too much information too soon the worker risks swamping the other person with data that are not heard or understood and will thus serve to confuse rather than inform.

(3) *Setting the 'contract' for the contact.* In many meetings with local people both they and the worker may want to discuss the terms on which the contact is taking place. The other person may want to know what use the worker is going to make of the outcomes of the contact (e.g. with whom is the information to be shared?) and be able to raise issues of confidentiality. The other person may wish to explore what he is 'being committed to' simply through the act of having a meeting with the worker. The worker may want to make it clear that she is not being committed to any course of action by virtue of talking with the other person about community issues.

(4) *Seeing the contact through.* This refers to the main body of the dicussion in which the worker seeks to achieve the goals that have been set for the contact. The worker asks questions, probes, stimulates reflection and discussion, throws in ideas and suggestions, establishes understanding with the other person, and integrates verbal communication with appropriate behavioural responses and cues. But the worker also listens and attends to what the other person is saying, trying to remember what she is

being told, and negotiating and clarifying the meaning of what is said.

The problem of remembering what has occurred in a contact is often a pressing one for workers in situations where it is not desirable or feasible to take notes or record on tape. Comprehensiveness and accuracy of what is remembered can be developed through training and experience. The following suggestions have been put forward as an aid to helping researchers doing participation observation to recall conversations:

look for 'key-words' in your subject's remarks;
concentrate on the first and last remarks in each conversation;
leave the setting as soon as you have observed as much as you can accurately remember;
make notes as soon after the contact as possible;
do not talk with anybody about the contact until you have made notes;
make your notes up after each contact, and do not wait until the end of the day to write up a number of contacts. (Taken from Bogdan and Taylor, 1975)

Recall can also be facilitated by endeavouring towards the end of the contact to summarise and clarify with the other person the major points that emerged in the discussion. This is also a way of reducing the risk of misrepresenting what has been said and agreed to between the worker and the other person.

It is also useful towards the end of the contact for the worker to focus more on consolidating his rapport with the other person than on pursuing the information he wants. This emphasis on rapport should help in providing the basis for further and continuing contacts with the other person.

After the Contact

The activities of the worker after the end of the contact seem to comprise the following:

recalling and writing up the contact – noting what has been obtained, areas discussed and points of agreement and disagreement. The worker might also record any further

135

action that may need to be taken as a result of the contact.

informing others of the contact or passing on ideas and information that is generated (where appropriate).

following up the contact – by sending (where appropriate) 'back-up' information about the worker and his interests; and encouraging the other person in any tasks he or she has agreed to do as a result of the contact.

We have already referred to the importance of taking note of the environment or setting in which contact-making is carried out. We want, too, to draw attention to the other kinds of environmental factors of which the worker ought to take account. Factors like the time of day and the weather, for example, will affect the success of contacts that a worker makes with people on a street or on their doorsteps. The 'culture' of an area, and particularly its attitudes to strangers and outsiders, will bear on a worker's attempts to make contact with local people. Other characteristics of an area such as its degree of 'closeness' and isolation have also been identified by workers as affecting their interventions.

The community workers modified their hopes after their first few visits to the estate. An early report of James' states that the Valley 'had a permanent air of depression' . . . It looks as if making initial contacts may be fairly difficult as it appears to be an isolated and close community. Other reports written by James at the time are full of words like 'isolated', 'apathetic' and 'rivalry'. The workers were told by residents that 'they would never get anything done here' and 'did they realise what the other people were like living in the area?' However, they persevered and visited all the houses on the estate. (Taylor *et al.*, 1976)

Thomas (1976b) has also described how the physical design of 'closed' and 'open' housing estates determines the type and quality of the worker's attempts to meet people and bring them together. We hope the reader will also consider how attempts at organising people are similarly influenced by other kinds of physical environments, particularly the layout and design of houses in estates, and the way factors like the horizontal or vertical patterning of roads, and the siting of amenities, may affect interchange between houses, streets and parts of a community.

Ways of Making Contact

It now seems appropriate to consider some of the different ways of initiating contacts with local people that are available to neighbourhood workers. The examples we give ought to be seen as illustrations, for we do not suggest that what we describe is comprehensive or that any of the techniques portrayed are necessarily right for all the situations in which workers find themselves. We would like our presentation of the different ways of making contact to be viewed in two lights: first, as an initial attempt to compile an inventory or repertoire of methods available, and from which the worker must judiciously choose for the purposes in hand; and, second, as an indication that most of the methods we describe are important areas in which practitioners should have some skill and confidence.

An important feature of the way neighbourhood workers initiate relationships with local people is that they will often 'reach out' to where the people are, taking the initiative and the first steps in making the contact. There are a number of reasons for this including the fact that neighbourhood workers do not ordinarily operate on the basis of referrals; and some communities may not be 'aware' of needs and the possibilities open to them through collective action. Often people will need help to understand and challenge the problems and forces that affect their lives. Even if *individuals* are aware of their needs, they may not perceive them as being the same as, or relating to, the problems of other individuals in the community.

There seem to be two aspects in the process of making local contacts, and it is a matter for the worker to judge whether they occur simultaneously or sequentially. In the first, the worker knows in advance who it is he wishes to see. He has a list of local people whom he sets out to meet. There are a number of ways in which this list will be compiled: the worker will have on it the names of officers of existing groups in the community; those who were interviewed whilst collecting data and expressed interest in the work or some issue or community problem; those mentioned by local people the worker 'ought' to see; and, finally, residents whose interest in a particular aspect of community affairs has been mentioned in the local newspapers and on deputations to the council. The worker may also have the names and addresses of people given by colleagues.

The second aspect of making contacts has to do with local people who are not 'known' or already affiliated to some grouping or organisation. In a sense, the worker wishes to reach out to, or to be reached by, the 'ordinary person in the street'. Depending on her approach, her method of contacting these people (i.e. the bulk of the population) will be haphazard and random and the people she will come into contact with will not be predictable. It is this second aspect of making contacts that we wish especially to examine further.

In order to do this it is helpful to conceive of a continuum formed by the question: who initiates the contact? At one end of the continuum we identify contacts initiated by the worker; at the other end, contacts initiated by residents. The distinction between worker- and resident-initiated contacts must be regarded as an aid to learning and as an attempt to impose some conceptual order on the array of opportunities open to the worker.

Contacts Initiated by the Worker

There are a variety of ways in which the worker can take the initiative and we describe some of these below.

Street Work   Here the street (or the square or yard in a block of flats) is the setting for the contact. The worker who is 'street working' has much in common with the kind of detached youth work described by Derek Cox in the Spitalfields area of London:

> I walk through Spitalfields, starting either at Liverpool Street or Cheshire Street. This has made me literally a 'street worker' talking to young people on street corners, on open spaces and in doorways. I drop in at cafes. This has proved to be a successful method of work as I meet many young people whilst zigzagging through Spitalfields. (1970)

Cox's account suggests some of the characteristics of street work for the neighbourhood worker. It may be done at its best when the weather is kind; streets may often not contain a cross-section of a community's population but only a part of it; the variety and quality of contacts will depend upon what kind of environment the street is part of (street work in Spitalfields, for instance, will be different from that on a long-established council estate in the north-east of England).

The purpose of street work is to gain information and get people interested in organising. One approach to this task is that of 'snow-balling' as described in the following reports by a worker wanting to organise block clubs.

> I first started out with the idea of organizing the whole area, and then I found out that this was ineffective. To do the job and get participation, you must do it on a small basis. You must organize block groups and then get the block groups to join together.
>
> To organize a block club, you go out on the street and you talk to one individual on the street and you ask him who has been doing what in the neighbourhood. Then he might express an interest himself. You also ask people that are standing around on the street what they want. It is important to find out if they want the street cleaned up, if they want a sewing club, and the like. Then you tell people that you talk to on the street that it is possible that other people have the same thoughts that they do about what they want and then ask them if it is possible to have a little group meeting on the block to find out how many people want the same things, and what they want. Then you get somebody working for you to develop that block. You try to get that person to have a little group meeting of her neighbors in her house. You need a person who will act as block leader right away so that she can take information from you to the people in her block. After she has had a block meeting, you try to get the five block leaders together in one group or section. I had actually selected the block leaders but I didn't think this was very good. (Ecklein and Lauffer, 1972)

This account describes a process of working with individuals who build up a nucleus of friends and neighbours around a particular interest.

An altogether different style is to work with people in aggregate on the street which becomes, in effect, the setting for meetings, discussion groups, theatre and other events that stimulate discussion and an interest in organising. A worker describes this approach on a council estate in Tynemouth.

We decided to test out the general level of feeling on the estate. To do this we planned a series of street meetings at which we would discuss with the tenants the problems. A leaflet was sent round to all the tenants outlining the reasons for the meeting and giving the dates, times and place in each of the streets where they would be held. On the day of each meeting another leaflet was distributed in each of the streets. We had already discussed this strategy with a number of tenants from the estate when they came into the project office for information. Before each meeting started we walked up and down the streets with a loud-hailer asking people to come out to the meeting. The pattern of the meeting was the same in each of the streets. By walking into the estate with a loud-hailer we roused their curiosity and at first small groups gathered up and down the street watched by others from their windows and front doors. As soon as we had got the groups together other tenants came out and joined the meeting. We had expected this initial reluctance to come out into the street and while we were going up and down the street we were involved in a number of good humoured exchanges about 'what the hell we were trying to do', and 'we've heard it all before'. By the time the meeting started there was on each occasion between thirty and fifty tenants involved. (Foster, 1975)

This is a helpful account, not least because it suggests a *planned and structured* approach to street work, particularly through the use of leaflets and the prior discussion of the strategy with some tenants. Attendance at the street meeting made less demands on participants than turning out to a 'traditional' public meeting; it also capitalised on people's affiliation to their street (rather than to the estate); and it benefited from the visibility of the event, that is, the meeting was an inclusive activity and residents may have been encouraged to attend by seeing that their neighbours were present.

The person who has done much to pave the way to a better understanding of the street in the urban environment is Jane Jacobs. Her book *The Death and Life of Great American Cities* is of value to neighbourhood workers in its understanding of the functions of the street in neighbourhood life. Her insights on the function of the street in promoting and controlling social interaction between residents, and between them and strangers, are a useful antidote to fears that the urban street is necessarily a hard, merciless place of confrontation and rejection.

Yet there are problems for the practitioner in street working. On the street his and her role is ambiguous; and people do appear to be rushing along pavements with great purpose, defying the worker to interrupt their pace and their thoughts. Some people, too, will outrightly reject an approach from a stranger, while others are suspicious and defensive about talking to someone they do not know. On the other hand, it is mostly the case that people are more friendly, interested and co-operative than they look! And there are ways in which the worker can help to reduce people's defensiveness. Some are described in the account of the Southwark Community Project, where the workers often found it better to adopt a passive role on the streets, creating opportunities and pretexts for others to initiate contact. Such opportunities were created through devices like standing at a bus stop, or carrying a street map, and looking uncertain about directions and places (Thomas, 1976).

There are three other aspects of street work that we have not mentioned yet. First, there is the use of pubs, cafes, shops, and so on, in which to meet people. Second, there is making contact with people at points where the worker knows they are to be found, for example, old age pensioners outside the post office on pension day, and in luncheon clubs; and claimants in and outside the local DHSS offices. Third, there is door-to-door knocking, in which the worker arrives 'cold' on the doorstep or has leafleted the houses in advance to say that she will be calling. The leaflet might say something about the worker, her agency and her interests in talking with local people. The information the worker puts on a leaflet about herself, and whether she uses a leaflet at all, will depend on her assessment of whether it will be helpful or not given what she knows about the neighbourhood.

Making contacts through knocking at doors may also be facilitated by an indirect approach. That is, the worker knocks on a door in order to distribute a leaflet or a community newspaper, waiting for views on the area to develop from more general discussion of the leaflet or newspaper. Indeed, the newspaper itself may be used to generate discussion if the worker draws attention to its contents. Finally, the worker who wishes to knock on doors

141

must consider how she will decide whose door to knock on. If she is unable to visit every household, then she must consider some kind of sample.

Video   The use of video equipment may be seen as another aspect of street working but it is sufficiently distinctive in its goals and technology to be treated separately. The most useful guide to the purposes, equipment and skills of video in community work is that produced by Inter-Action (1975). There are, however, few case studies from practitioners about their use of video. The following account of the use of video, which also describes its value in situations other than contact-making, is taken from the Inter-Action handbook.

Apart from its 'instant television' quality, an advantage of video is the ease with which anyone can be taught how to use it. The controls on the camera and recorder are extremely simple and easy to operate. Anyone can be trained to be reasonably competent within half-an-hour. In addition, the tape is relatively cheap, and most important, it can be erased and used many times, giving a picture quality approximately the same as that on a television as seen at home. Basically, then, video is a cheap, immediate, easy-to-use recording device. But the critical factor in video's success as an organising tool is its ability to create a dialogue and bring people together.

The very fact of making such a powerful tool available to people often accomplishes a great deal by building self-confidence in their ability to speak for themselves and present their own cases. It is often this 'process' that people go through in producing a videotape that is much more important than the resulting 'product'. By mastering the use of technical equipment, they gain confidence individually. By pinpointing issues relevant in their area, they clarify common overriding problems. By beginning to work together (and video is very much a team effort) and actually doing something tangible, they may form a strong active unit. One community worker in Lambeth had to work hard to convince a group of tenants that making a tape to assist in the formation of a tenants' association was worth doing. In the end, they really enjoyed making the tape, began to cohere as a group though not without problems, and went on to form the core of a strong tenants' association to replace a weak and disheartened one.

Video can have a significant 'welding' or catalysing effect on community action.

The search for evidence to back up a case requires that the group goes out into the community to interview people and record conditions. Video makes it easier to approach strangers, legitimising discussion in the same way as a man-in-the-street interview. However, it should be noted here – and it cannot be overemphasised – that video is only a tool. It can only reflect issues relevant to the people who use it. It can act as a focus for people, but the human dimension always remains the most important element. Video is not a substitute for personal contact and communication, but is an extension of it. How then can video be used in specific ways to promote community activities?

AS AN INFORMATION TOOL   At its simplest level, it can be used as a source of information about events and activities occurring in the neighbourhood. Organisations can use the equipment to produce programmes about what they are doing. This could serve either to attract more participants or members or simply to make residents aware of the kind of services or opportunities that are available, ranging from welfare and housing rights to the structure of local government. These can be played back at meetings of local groups, in the market place, in community houses or even in local pubs.

AS A 'TRIGGER' TAPE   An extension of the basic information tape is the 'tripper tape' designed not only to inform people, but also to raise their level of awareness and stimulate action on any given issue. The mere presence of a group of mothers on an estate using a video camera and asking questions about the bad housing conditions will usually arouse an interest in the issue among other residents. Experience has also shown that a visual presentation of an issue rather than a verbal or written report is much more effective. Everyone on the estate may have *heard* that Mrs Brown's ceiling is falling in, but when it is *seen* on TV the effect is quite different.

AS A WAY OF GETTING PEOPLE TO MEETINGS   Video has a novelty value that will draw people to 'yet another meeting'. It is a 'telly programme' made by local people, relating directly to them and their community. People come to see themselves, their kids or their neighbours on TV and, more important, they will stay on to discuss the points raised by the programme.

AS A WAY OF SHOWING COMMON PROBLEMS AND CONCERNS   Video has proved instrumental in bringing both individuals and groups together by demonstrating that they share common concerns or situations. Whether it be problems of housing, education or employment or situations common to certain groups within the community, such as children, young wives or pensioners, video can be used to show that the experiences that individuals face are common problems shared by others. This process may in turn lead to a discussion of possible avenues for collective action.

AS A WAY OF ILLUSTRATING OTHER SUCCESSFUL ACTIONS   On a wider scale, video can be used to link groups, geographically separate, but closely related by a common situation. Being able to show a group a tape about another group somewhere else with a similar problem, and showing the methods that were used to overcome that problem, often stimulates the viewers to attempt similar actions. To see that something has been done successfully elsewhere is a positive factor in the development of many groups and projects.

AS A NEW FORM OF PRESENTING INFORMATION TO AUTHORITIES Video can perform a powerful function when used in meetings with officials or experts. A videotape can often give 'ordinary' people a sense of self-confidence by putting their case in a coherent and well-thought-out form. In this way, video provides an effective voice to people who might not be given a proper hearing when other more conventional tactics such as letters, telephone calls and even delegations have failed. This has often been illustrated by groups of children using video to present their case concerning a lack of play facilities to both adult tenants' associations and the local authority. An additional and very real advantage of video is its ability to allow a group to present a case coherently and in its entirety. This will prevent experienced politicians and officials from interrupting the group and causing it to lose the thread of its argument.

AS A WAY OF EXAMINING THE DEVELOPMENT OF THE GROUP
Because of its ability to provide immediate playback, video can
enable a group to examine its own progress and development.
Group discussions and activities can be recorded and immediately
shown to the participants, either adults or children, often forcing
them to analyse the way in which they react to others. This self-
awareness is of benefit to both the individual and the group in that
barriers to communication can be identified and dealt with. On a
more practical level, this kind of self-examination could lead to
role play situations dealing with the particular experience of any
group.

AS ENTERTAINMENT As a sheer entertainment medium, video is
invaluable. Whether it is used to document the local festival for
playback during the year or to record a 'Kung Fu' programme
enacted on the local adventure playground, it provides people
with a further opportunity to take an interest in their community
and their neighbours.

AS A CLOSED-CIRCUIT FACILITY IN THE MARKET OR SHOP FRONT
Video offers a unique experience – closed-circuit TV. Children
and adults alike are thrilled to see their own image on TV. A
closed-circuit set-up on a street information stall or in a shop
window can act as a visual magnet to draw people, who can then
be presented with detailed information, using video and printed
material, on a neighbourhood issue. (Inter-Action, 1975. The
handbook is available from 14 Talacre Road, London NW5.)
   There are of course limitations and difficulties in using video,
and these are also discussed in the handbook. It can be used
indiscriminately, and with ill-defined objectives and planning. The
showing back of video needs adequate preparation and facilities,
and often the poor quality of the tape (particularly its sound) will
detract from its impact.

Probes: or Flying Kites in the Community The idea of 'probes' is
found in Tom Lovett's account of his adult education work in
Liverpool. Probes were part of a larger strategy to make contact
with local people that Lovett describes as the exploration,
investigation and experiment phase of his early work (1975). The
initiation of these probes was a reflection of the limited scope

145

offered to the adult educator for getting in touch with parents through schools.

The probes were 'project-initiated exercises in adult education' whose purpose was both to make contacts with local people and to test their assumptions about and reactions to adult education. The probes were a project on the history of a neighbourhood run in a local school; an exhibition of the work of seven schools in a department store; and an 'informal' neighbourhood survey 'to "chat people up" and discover the whole range of interests and problems'.

Neighbourhood workers have used other kinds of probes such as welfare rights stalls, advice sessions, playschemes and festivals. While these provide a valuable service in their own right, they also allow the worker to enter the community in a purposive way and thus establish contact with local people. The issues or ideas around which the probes are organised may not reflect the most pressing concerns of the worker or neighbourhood – indeed, probes are valuable because these concerns may not even be known to the worker, but the probe provides a way of coming to know them.

The Survey The legitimisation of the worker's contacts is a theme that has appeared several times in this chapter, whether in regard to video, the use of leaflets when door-knocking, or probes. The survey is likewise a device that legitimates the worker's activities:

> One advantage of using a questionnaire survey is that at the initial point of contact it gives the worker what is becoming a universally recognised and largely accepted role. For some reason people will talk to someone on their door-step who says he is doing a survey when they might be much more reluctant to get into conversation without this explanation of his presence. (Baldock, 1974)

We have already discussed surveys and self-surveys in the chapter on data collection, and referred readers to considerations and references that will help to ensure that surveys are done with proper care and regard to the principles of social research methods. Such propriety was important because the purpose of the survey was to gather valid and reliable information on which a worker's decisions could be made. But in this stage, the worker is considering a survey primarily to make contact with people. The survey is a recruiting device and one to raise consciousness about an issue in an area. As such, argues Baldock, 'it need not be subject to the same criteria as a sociologically respectable survey would be, and its findings cannot be used as though it were such a survey'.

Some of the ways in which a contact-making survey differs from the 'sociologically respectable' kind are contained in the following account of a survey by a community worker:

Together, staff members and volunteers from each building or building complex interviewed someone in each apartment in that building. We asked similar questions everywhere, but we put the stress on certain issues in each place. For example, with the old folks we focused more on questions dealing with transportation and with muggings. With mothers of young kids we focused on child-care need and on the broken washing machines.

The canvassers who went from door to door did not just ask questions and leave. They stayed and talked – about anything people had on their minds, and about why we were there in the project. A 20-minute interview could easily stretch into an hour. It was never time wasted. We identified potential leaders, located the disinterested, and got insights into the politics of the housing authority. Most important, we began establishing communication links – not just between ourselves and the people – but among them too. Bringing residents along and having them do some of the canvassing was very helpful. They were able to dispel some of the mistrust people showed strangers. On the other hand, sometimes people in the apartments were not prepared to open up and tell one neighbor about a problem they were having with another neighbor. So there are some disadvantages too.

Sometimes you get information that could never have come out in a formal survey, and we shared this information rather purposefully. Like, we would tell Mrs Cooley on the sixth floor that Mrs Robinson on the third had had the same trouble with her sink and how she managed to maneuver through the bureaucracy to get it fixed. We gave her Mrs Robinson's phone number so she could get the whole story. (Ecklein and Lauffer, 1972)

Surveys are also used by neighbourhood workers at the later phase of the neighbourhood process, 'forming and building an organisation', and we discuss surveys in this context in the next chapter.

The Petition   The collecting of signatures for a petition can serve many purposes: it can support a demand made by a local group of decision-makers; and gain publicity for a group and spread information about the issues with which it is concerned. It is also an aid to organising by attracting new recruits to a group, and possibly other resources such as finance. And for the worker the petition is also a way into a neighbourhood in order to make contact with people and learn more about community issues. A petition carried out by the worker with one or two community residents can lead to the formation of a small group of interested people.

Most of the strategies we have discussed so far lead sooner or later to the worker meeting local residents in a small group. In one sense, then, the small group is part of these other strategies, and perhaps does not need to be treated separately. On the other hand, it represents an approach to making contacts and organising that is distinctive if only because the worker uses it to *meet* other people. The host of the group meeting will have invited residents whom the worker has not previously met. This is different from other strategies we have described when the worker meets as a group people he has already been in contact with individually. The following account indicates the process of using small groups in order to build up community contact:

The organizer next will begin to relate the newly concretized vision to the problems and grievances of the poor. He may seek invitations to informal 'house meetings'. At each he will begin discussions by briefly describing his work to a small group of neighbors, friends or relatives of the hosts, using illustrations of the accomplishments of the organized poor in other places. He mentions the legitimators who will have agreed to vouch for him. Very early the organizer attempts to elicit from persons at the meeting their ideas of what needs to be done and which could possibly be done through collective action.

These are *agitational* qustions since they raise the possibility of doing something about aspects of reality which are normally regarded fatalistically . . .

At the end of the house meeting the organizer gets the names, addresses and telephone numbers of those persons who have attended, and seeks invitations from them to hold other house meetings in their houses with other guests present. In this way an organizer works his way along informal lines of communication in the area and begins a redefinition of the situation and a first awareness of the possibility of forming an organization of the poor. Even if he works at top speed, attending two or more house meetings each day, it will take many weeks for the organizer to talk with the largest possible number of people in the area. In the meantime the house meeting drive may have run into many hitches. For example, persons who agree to have a house meeting may change their minds and the organizer will find no-one at home when he arrives. In some cases enemies of organizations will spread rumors which frighten people away from the idea that they can organize . . .

At the time which seems most favorable, a meeting will be held to which everyone in the area has been invited. At this meeting the poor will officially begin to form their organization. Through an analogous process, over a larger area in which there are enough existing organizations with mass support, the organizer will later bind together many organizations of the poor into an organization-of-organizations. (Haggstrom, 1969)

The Public Meeting The public meeting is almost always an essential step in group development and organisation. It is through the public meeting that a constituency usually elects its comittee, decides on a constitution and gives the committee a mandate from which to work. It is through the public meeting that grievances can be aired, officials confronted and the collective dimensions of a problem made manifest to individuals. In this section, however, we want only to consider the public meeting *as a way of initially contacting people*, and we will leave discussion of its other functions as described above until the next chapter.

The worker using the public meeting as a contacting or recruiting mechanism will typically work by herself or with some residents in putting around some posters and leaflets announcing the meeting, its agenda and where it is to be held. Such work will be preceded by a minimum of contact-making using other strategies as outlined above; in effect, the public meeting is called cold. A criticism of this kind of approach has already been made by one of the authors (Thomas, 1976), who sees the public meeting 'as the outcome of preliminary efforts at intervention by the community worker rather than as a mechanism that is useful by itself as a way of identifying and recruiting members to its work . . . we suspect . . . that the probabilities of success in using a public meeting as the initial means of contact are not great'. Jacobs has also cautioned that:

> The emergence of a local leadership is a complex process, dependent upon the personalities and issues involved, existing social relationships, chance and not least of all, the influence of the community workers. It is usually a mistake for outsiders to attempt to initiate a local organization simply by calling a public meeting in the belief that leaders will come forward. It is as likely as not to result in the formation of a non-representative group with the one middle-class resident being elected as chairman. (1976)

What are the factors that make for a successful public meeting? The following seem to be important, though they can all be set at nought by bad weather that persuades people to stay at home.

(1) *Choose the right issue* People will turn out if the issue is salient for them, and presented to them in a concrete and relevant way. Abstract descriptions of an issue will encourage people to stay at home; 'What's in it for me?' will be a question in many people's minds when deciding whether or not to turn out. 'What can *we* do about it?' is another question – the callers of the meeting will have to show some indication of the possibilities for change that can be explored if people take the first step and come to the meeting.

(2) *Provide inducement to come* Some form of entertainment is a useful inducement; so, too, is the showing of a film relevant to the issue and the presence of video and television cameras.

(3) *Attend to detail in advertising and recruitment* There should be both face-to-face contact with residents personally invited to come, and encouraged to bring friends and neighbours,

as well as the use of posters, leaflets and the media to reach a larger number of people.

Reminders about the meeting are essential – leaflets should be distributed in advance of the meeting, the week of the meeting and some hours before it. If enough manpower is available people should be personally reminded through door-knocking on the evening of the meeting, and 'fetched' to the meeting if they have expressed interest but seemed shy or diffident about attending. Another useful form of reminder is to hold a video session in the morning or afternoon, letting people know it will be shown at the meeting. Remember, too, that it can be more effective to recruit people to a meeting by going through existing networks, groups, clubs and so forth than by the 'cold' leafletting of houses and flats.

(4) *Specify goals in advance* Work out beforehand what the meeting is supposed to achieve, and how this will be done. Make arrangements beforehand if you expect people to do things immediately after the meeting – it's no good asking for volunteers to put some leaflets around after the meeting if the leaflets are not available.

(5) *Plan the meeting carefully* The venue must be convenient and acceptable to most of the residents, as must the day and time of the meeting (check the television programmes and football fixtures before deciding day and time!). The size of the room is important – not so large that although there has been a good turn-out it *looks* small and discourages residents; and not so small that people are uncomfortable and irritated. Seating arrangements must be thought about – is the arrangement of the audience in ranked chairs confronted by a platform of speakers the most effective? Foster has described, for instance, an arrangement of concentric circles though the tenants subsequently changed it (1975). Work out the programme carefully, ensuring some way of keeping speakers to their time limits – and is it necessary for the meeting to spend the whole time as a large group? Finally, think about briefing 'stooges' to ask questions or to volunteer at the right time in order to get the meeting rolling.

In areas hit hard by unemployment, workers are turning to day-time meetings rather than evening ones. Day meetings are also more likely to be effective in neighbourhoods where residents' fear of crime inhibits their involvement in community activities after dark.

Mediated Contacts   We use the term mediated contacts to refer to the those situations where some third party or event or item brings together the worker and some local residents. The fact that this occurs will often be at the initiative of the worker, so we consider it appropriate to discuss these contacts within this section.

Mediated contacts often provide through the action of the third party an external legitimisation both of the worker's role and interest, and of his or her activity in seeking out local people to talk with them. It is not assumed, however, that this legitimisation will necessarily be helpful to the neighbourhood worker; being introduced to residents by a third party who is not well regarded may both legitimate and impair the worker's attempts to get to know local people and issues. It may also be difficult to get a conversation going with someone in the presence of a third party – perhaps the worker needs to say 'hello' casually and arrange an appointment alone with the person.

We wish to mention only some of the more common or traditional kinds of mediated contacts. These appear to include the following.

THE GATE-KEEPER OR GO-BETWEEN   The neighbourhood worker is often able to make contacts with local people through introductions made by other residents, councillors and other professionals in the neighbourhood. Each kind of go-between – whether it be a shop-keeper, social worker, resident, caretaker or whoever – will carry its own costs and benefits to the worker. Her skill is in being able to perceive and mobilise the go-betweens that are most appropriate for each of the contacts that she wishes to make. To do this the worker needs some knowledge of the community and the relationships between different people and roles within it. Hence the go-between may be most safely used when the worker has begun to find her way around the community, and not in the early stages of intervention. People who act as go-betweens may also require something (e.g. information, support for a proposal) from the worker in return; the cost of giving this has to be accounted for when deciding whether or not to use a go-between.

GOING THROUGH EXISTING ORGANISATIONS   This way of making contacts is perhaps a special aspect of the use of a go-between.

Lovett describes how links with organisations such as schools, a community council, a church, the Shelter Neighbourhood Action Project, community centres and a community arts project each opened up contacts with local people (1975). McGrath describes how contact was made with a local Asian community by working through and with the Muslim Welfare Society (1975a). Two other contributors to the volume in which the McGrath paper appears write about making contacts and organising people through the use of defunct or fading community groups (Foster and Green, 1975).

As with more personal go-betweens, the choice of going through one organisation rather than another predetermines the kinds of contacts the worker will make, and the kinds of issues presented to her. One wonders, for instance, about the differences there would have been in attempting to contact Asian immigrants if this had been done through the local community relations committee rather than the Muslim Welfare Society.

The kind of organisations through which one might make contacts may have little to do with the worker's goals. Lovett, for instance, describes how he got to know local people by 'becoming involved in a number of community activities which, on the surface at least, bore no relationship to adult education'.

BY REFERRAL   Local people may be referred to the worker by staff in her own or other agencies. This might occur, for example, because an individual client comes from the area in which it is known that the community worker is interested; or the caseworker perceives that her client's 'problem' has a collective basis and can best be dealt with through collective action.

PUBLIC INFORMATION SOURCES   Here the worker is able to contact people through the 'mediation' of, for example, a newspaper story or a planning application. The worker might read of some named tenants in a local paper who are concerned about some aspect of their estate; and take this report as an invitation to seek them out and express her interests in learning more about their concerns. Thomas has also provided an example of work initiated by a notice about a public inquiry on the side of a building (1976).

Contacts Initiated by Residents

Resident-initiated contacts occur when a worker has been established in an area. He may have spent some time making contacts through ways described in the previous section, started to work with local groups, and become known in the neighbourhood as a person whom people can ask for certain kinds of advice and help. As his work and interests become better known, he will be approached by residents and invited to discuss an issue or problem around which some local people will have already come together. Such an existing group may look to the worker for help in forming themselves into an organisation; for specific resources that they need to carry out their work more effectively; or for advice on some particular aspect of their activities such as the procedures for urban aid funding or the address of a committee chairman.

The type of concerns that residents will thus bring to a worker will partly be determined by their perception of his responsibilities and skills as they have been defined by his work with existing groups in the community; by their understanding of the remit of his employing agency; and by accounts of his work and usefulness that have been disseminated along the community's informal information networks. The worker will therefore also have to negotiate *mis*understandings about his role and relevance as a resource, and to respond to requests for help that are not in line with his own (or his agency's) priorities, skills, values, and so on.

Residents will also approach a worker as a result of some event or incident in the community that brings them together or highlights a salient issue or problem. For example, unfavourable press publicity about an estate may precipitate the formation of a tenants' association.

In this part of the chapter, however, we want to deal with other kinds of resident-initiated contacts that are associated with the earlier phases of the worker's intervention. The distinguishing characteristic of this approach to contact-making is that the neighbourhood worker purposefully creates opportunities for local people to make the first contact and to take the initiative in defining an area of interest or concern. The worker 'sits back' and waits for residents to come to him; the onus is placed on residents to make use of the services that are placed at the disposal of residents, usually without much publicity and explanation. We wish in particular to examine two broad categories of resident-initiated contacts, namely, *imbricated or overlapping roles* and the development of *advice centres*.

Imbricated Roles   Here the worker has a role in the neighbourhood other than that of worker. He has a status or position that is additional to that of neighbourhood worker. Perhaps the best known of imbricated neighbourhood roles is that of the worker who is also a resident in the neighbourhood in which she is working. As a consequence, she begins to make her contact with residents, and they with her as a resident; in this way her position as a resident is one that facilitates opportunities for residents to initiate contact with her, sometimes relating to her as a resident, sometimes as a worker.

It is the worker-resident imbrication that we want to look at further in this section; but there are also other imbrications such as the worker who is also an employee of a local group(s); and the neighbourhood worker who has also another established professional role in the area such as a priest or teacher. These, too, may be seen as affording opportunities for resident-initiated contacts.

Whether one should live in the neighbourhood that one works in has been an issue of perennial discussion in community work. It is argued, on the one hand, that living in an area brings the worker familiarity with all aspects of its life, is an expression of commitment to and identification with it, and provides a 'natural' way for residents to get to know the services and resources the worker can offer. It helps to overcome suspicion or distrust of outsiders and hostility to those who are perceived to commute into areas of disadvantage in order 'to do good works'. It is also suggested that residence offers one of the few ways of being responsive to events and demands in the community as they arise – problems do not confine themselves to the hours between nine and five. Neighbourhood workers will also value the satisfaction to themselves that comes of living in the neighbourhood they work in, and of being close to where the action is. Residence may be seen, too, as helping the worker to avoid importing 'outside' values and perspectives into the work in the neighbourhood.

On the other hand, it is suggested that while living in the area does have considerable benefits, it asks too much of the worker's time and energies. It blurs the boundary between work and non-work and exposes the worker to being always 'on call' to deal with group and individual problems. Besides sapping the worker of energy and interest, being on call in this way may also work against the interests of the neighbourhood. It may foster overdependence on the worker as a resource and undermine the usefulness of other local people in dealing with community issues; indeed, it may push the worker into the role of community leader. The worker is also at risk of getting too involved in neighbourhood affairs, particularly in sectional conflicts and disputes from which she should be able to distance herself in order to facilitate the work of a neighbourhood group. It is also pointed out that the family situation of some workers (e.g. a spouse tied to work in some other neighbourhood) as well as other factors like the scarcity of suitable accommodation often make it impracticable for the worker to take up residence. A worker might also feel reluctant both to expose her family to the demands of being 'on call' and to take up living accommodation that might be needed more by other local families.

It is clear that there are arguments for and against taking up residence in a neighbourhood; our concern here is largely to point out that residence is one of the important ways in which resident-initiated contacts may be developed. We want also to suggest that the imbrication of resident and worker roles may be best seen as a continuum, and that the point on the continuum occupied by any worker – that is, to what extent he takes up the respective roles of worker and resident – is a matter of decision in the light of factors like the characteristics of the neighbourhood and what the worker wishes to achieve.

The continuum of roles runs from that of Complete Resident, through the Resident-as-Worker, the Worker-as-Resident, to the Complete Worker. (This analysis is inspired by Raymond Gold's work, 1969, on roles in participant observation.)

THE COMPLETE RESIDENT   In its extreme form this is a role of pretence. The worker takes up residence in the area he will work in, and does not reveal to residents his employment or his interest in community work, and his aspiration to work with them in some kind of collective organising effort. He takes part in local groups as a resident and the participants know him in no other role. He may live on supplementary benefit, have a part-time job or take an occupation (like a milkman) that gives him time to do his organising work. In principle, this type of work might be financed by a voluntary or statutory agency, and the worker also conceals this fact from local people.

The role of complete resident may also be seen as one that the worker takes up in the early phase of his residence in a neighbourhood, before he has explained his community work role or before it has been mentioned by local residents. The worker may also choose to delay informing people of his community work role because he thinks that to do so would be to prejudice his long-term organising efforts. Such a decision was taken by workers who moved into a rural area and initially presented themselves only as staff members of a distant university. They held back information on their organising intentions because their predecessors, who had been more explicit, 'were arrested on sedition charges, thrown into jail, and investigated by the McCellan Committee. Their library was stolen, and their house was bombed. We didn't want that to happen to us. Above all, we did not want to be singled out as outside trouble-makers' (Ecklein and Lauffer, 1972). The workers set up house in an old school and it was through the process of getting it suitable for habitation that they gradually got to know the local people.

THE RESIDENT-AS-WORKER At this point in the continuum the person's role in the neighbourhood is primarily that of a resident. The worker might primarily *see* and identify herself as a resident first, and a worker second, as described by Ilys Booker: 'My first role is that of a resident in the area, using the services as all residents do and extending my connections with individuals and groups as I become familiar to people' (in Mitton and Morrison, 1972). But Booker was also aware of the limitations of the resident-as-worker role, for she wrote:

> There is first the question of how one is viewed by members of the community. If one is merely a householder resident in the area, even if one states from time to time why one is there, it is most unlikely that anyone will come asking for something to be done. This is not only because this method of working ... is

little known, but because it is in the very nature of neighbour-hood life that relationships of any depth take long months, and often years, to mature.

The resident-as-worker role is more usually thrust upon a worker by an event or issue that crops up in the area in which he is living, and which may not be the area in which he is doing his community work. John Benington describes the resident-as-worker role in his case study of Gosford Green Residents' Association where he writes about grievances in the neighbour-hood, some of which 'affected our own family life, and so I began to talk with some of my neighbours about the possibility of organised action to tackle the situation effectively' (1975).

Other examples of the resident-as-worker are provided by the part-time worker who lives in the area he works in; and by the local resident who has become a community worker in the neighbourhood in which he lives. His friends and neighbours may continue to relate primarily to him as a resident, not wanting to accept, or unable to understand, the nature of his new community work role.

THE WORKER-AS-RESIDENT   This is the more common role where the neighbourhood worker decides to live in the area in which she has been employed to work. She is probably seen primarily as an outsider whose interests and services are at first difficult to grasp, but later emerge as a helpful contribution to group activity. The worker believes that her status as a resident helps her to become better known to local people, and they are more able to understand and use her assistance. We have already discussed the pros and cons of this role. There appear to be many examples of the role in British community work practice, and some accounts of community work from this role are to be found in the literature (see, for example, Lovett, 1975).

THE COMPLETE WORKER   With this role, the neighbourhood worker does not make use of her residence in the neighbourhood to facilitate her contact-making and attempts at organising. She may be living in the area reluctantly, and she places extremely tight boundaries between her work and her home and social life. The majority of her contacts with local people are in the context of her community work, and not her resident, role. It is perhaps difficult to imagine that this would prove to be an effective role for a community worker. However, it might be a role that characterises the ending phase of a worker's intervention as she prepares to end work in the neighbourhood. She may well decide to reduce all social and non-work contacts with residents as part of her planned withdrawal. This is discussed more fully in Chapter 10 on endings in neighbourhood work.

The final point we wish to make about residence in the area of work is that the kinds of contacts that are made, and the type and quality of information gathered, will vary with particular phases of residence. This is almost a truism: the worker's contacts and information at the point of first moving into a community are likely to be different from those when he is a firmly established resident.

We now want to leave the imbrication of worker and resident roles and turn to another kind of activity in neighbourhood work that facilitates resident-initiated contacts.

Advice Centres and Projects   Opening up an advice centre or neighbourhood project, or running an advice service from some other base such as a stall or mobile van, allows people to take the initiative in bringing to workers issues (perhaps personally defined at first) that may form the basis of collective neighbourhood action. Because the function of these centres and projects is relatively well understood there may be fewer or different problems for the workers, as compared with contacts they initiate themselves, about introducing themselves and establishing the kinds of services they have to offer. They can work with people who present themselves, consider action on their presenting issues, and they in turn can relate to the workers as advice-givers; in so doing the workers can gain acceptance and credibility and begin to put forward their other skills and interest in organising for collective action.

Of course, neighbourhood workers in such centres may also use techniques described in the earlier section that give them the initiative in making contacts with local people. In addition, an advice centre can decide upon what degree of outreach it wishes to adopt in encouraging people to come to the centre. Leissner (1967) has described the degrees of outreach or 'aggressiveness' that an advice centre can decide upon. It may simply open up for business with no publicity in an accessible location; or publicise its services through the newspapers, posters, circulars to residents, and letters to community organisations and service agencies; or, more aggressively still, knock on doors in order to explain its services to local people.

A localised advice/information centre or neighbourhood project may seem an effective base from which to offer services; they are not, however, without their problems and these have been discussed in several accounts by practitioners (for example, Bond, 1975; Hatch *et al.*, 1977; Butcher, 1976) who indicate that among the important issues that determine the effectiveness of a centre or project are the following:

THE NATURE OF RECEPTION FACILITIES   Bond suggests that initially a highly qualified, high-status worker is needed to do reception to take seriously and precisely the problem an individual is presenting; because first impressions created through 'counter staff' lay the basis for the way the whole agency is perceived and responded to; and because reception staff need also to be able to see the public aspects of individuals' problems that may lend themselves to collective action.

THE NATURE OF RESPONDING TO PROBLEMS   A centre has to be seen to be taking action and doing something of value to individual callers. It has to establish a reputation for getting things done. But Bond has suggested that this will or may produce an advocacy style of intervention on behalf of individuals that not only undermines attempts to get individuals to do things for themselves, but also the efforts of the worker to alert people to the need to deal with problems collectively. Whilst the advice centre works well in creating opportunities for contact between workers and residents the end-purpose of this contact-making (i.e. to organise for collective action) may be jeopardised if the centre's style of response to individual problems encourages dependency and a feeling of satisfaction with an individual definition of, and solution to, a problem.

HOW TO DEAL WITH INDIVIDUAL INQUIRIES THAT FALL OUTSIDE THE REMIT OF THE CENTRE OR PROJECT   It may not be part of a centre's remit to respond to an individual's private or family problems and emergencies that might be more the concern of social services agencies. The centre may not want to take on 'casework' of this kind and what is crucial is the *manner* in which it avoids doing this kind of work. It will not want to acquire a reputation of 'turning people away' or 'not being interested in people's problems'; if it refers individuals to other agencies, it also runs the risk of making people feel fobbed off.

AN INITIAL AND SOMETIMES CONTINUING CONFUSION ABOUT THE CENTRE'S ROLE, and an identification of the centre with other agencies such as the social services, the housing department, and the social security.

MAKING THE CENTRE ACCESSIBLE Workers will be frustrated in their efforts to make contact with local people if their premises are badly sited, and their appearance such that it deters people from entering. The great care that is needed in making a centre accessible is indicated in the following account of the Hillfields Information and Opinion Centre in Coventry (Bond, 1975). The workers were motivated to 'attract as many callers as possible' so they wanted the centre to be 'as accessible as possible both geographically and psychologically'. The worker writes:

> To meet these conditions, a shop was selected in the middle of the main shopping street of the area and deliberately designed to be as unlike a formal council office as possible, both in physical appearance and style of operation. It was possible to see through the plate-glass window of the shop into a pleasant carpeted room furnished with a settee and several armchairs, and a desk set informally at an angle in the corner. The downstairs room of the shop was divided by a sliding partition so that private telephone calls or interviews could take place in the back of the shop. A small kitchen and lavatory were situated next to the downstairs room, and cups of tea were constantly available . . . it was decided not to use the word 'advice' in the name of the centre to counteract any assumption that the problems of the neighbourhood necessarily lay in the residents who therefore needed to be given 'advice'. It was also thought that for someone to come through a door labelled 'Advice Centre' they would to some extent have to define themselves as

someone with a 'problem', and that this would be a great disadvantage in attempting to attract as wide a cross-section of local residents as possible.

This account highlights the importance of producing for the centre an image and an atmosphere that is conducive to contact-making and the development of work with groups. The ingredients of this image/atmosphere are not only to do with the informality and friendliness of the centre, and the quality of the concern of the workers in an individual's problems; they are also to do with the social relationships that are developed between the centre's workers, and between them and the users of the centre. The absence or minimum of hierarchical relationships and procedures between staff, and between staff and users, and the insistence on a more collegiate and participatory milieu contribute to making a centre an accessible resource.

THE TYPES OF WORKERS   There seem to be two issues here, both of which influence a centre's effectiveness for contact-making and organising. The first is about whether, and at what stage, a centre is staffed (and managed) by professional workers and/or by local residents; and the second is the nature of relationships between the specialist and the generalist worker in a centre, something which seems to be especially salient in law and welfare rights centres.

The involvement of local people in running and managing a centre or project is rightly an important value in neighbourhood work. Participation is valued in its own right and because it contributes substantially towards achieving the process or educational aims of neighbourhood workers. But a word of caution: the participation of local people in a project or centre may become so sanctified a value that it inhibits workers from asking further crucial questions. What is to be achieved by involving local people? What are the goals to which participation is a means? Can these goals be achieved by participation? Are there more effective ways of attaining them? The pragmatic as well as the normative aspects of participation must be addressed by the workers in each centre.

The workers in the Hillfields centre found very persuasive practical and political reasons for handing over the centre to residents – it would provide an opportunity for them to exercise some control over their own lives and local resources; to develop their own style of operating the centre; to create an independent centre to change policies and procedures of service agencies and to provide a more effective advocacy service; and to increase the possibility that the centre would remain in existence after the CDP had finished.

This account of some considerations relevant to the setting up and running of advice centres does not comprise a comprehensive discussion of the role and function of centres. We have attempted to review only some of those factors about such centres and projects that are pertinent to our discussion of advice centres as a mechanism through which resident-initiated contacts are made possible.

Conclusions

Our purpose in this chapter has been to indicate the importance of contact-making, the functions it serves and the several forms that it may take. We are aware that in describing the forms we have elaborated upon methods and techniques in a way that may suggest to the reader an over-mechanistic view of the worker's tasks in making contacts with people. We accept that this may be a cost of our presentation of the material in this chapter, but it is one that we decided to bear in order to make clear the repertoire of methods at the disposal of the worker.

We do not, however, want to lose sight of the worker (or local people, for that matter) nor to underestimate the contributions to the success of contact-making of other, sometimes intangible, factors like the worker's stamina, enthusiasm and personal abilities to relate to a variety of individuals and groups.

One of the distinctive themes in this chapter has been *choice* – choosing the kind of approach to making contacts in the light of relevant factors such as the worker's own skills and confidence, and the physical and social character of the community. A choice has to be made in order to optimise the worker's opportunities for *communication* with local people, and the kind of communication that will help achieve greater understanding of the community and better rapport with its residents.

We have emphasised the careful choosing and planning of the means of communication, not only to draw attention to the purposeful way in which the worker might take up the tasks of contact-making, but also to caution workers against resorting to means of contact-making without appraising those most suitable for particular circumstances. It is often too easy to resort to ways of doing things that are well tried; that one feels comfortable with; that are conveniently at hand; or that were tried 'last time'. These are sound criteria for choice only if the worker is satisfied that the methods chosen are *also* right for the situation he or she presently faces.

CHAPTER 6

Forming and Building Organisations

From Group to Organisation
  Community conditions
  Community issues
Forming an Organisation
  Checking feasibility and
  desirability
  Encouraging leadership
  Early help
  Anticipating
  'One thing leads to another'

Surveys
Motivations of group members
The wider constituency
Clear goals
Building an Organisation
  Organisational structure
  Tactics and strategies
  Group cohesion
Public Meetings

When moving to an examination of community organising, the extent of documentation and commentary becomes noticeably richer. One thinks, for example, of some of Alinsky's most potent writing, particularly in *Reveille for Radicals* (1969), and of the work done by Rothman and his associates (1976) on 'field test' experiences of community workers.

In this country, the number of published accounts of workers' successes and failures when organising groups has grown steadily, as has the literature which describes and analyses community projects. There is also a widespread existence of good quality mimeograph material, some of which circulates within limited networks of interested persons, a sort of *samizdat* outlet for neighbourhood work which allows workers to share, test out and benefit from others' experiences. Neighbourhood work in this sense is in a phase of development more akin to producing rushes for inspection, acceptance or rejection than to submitting ordered material ready for the cutting room.

In our model of the neighbourhood work process we are entering that part of practice which typically embodies the 'stuff' or nuts and bolts of the neighbourhood worker's role. In this chapter we concentrate on the area of forming and giving strength to community groups. Then, in the following three chaptres, we shall explore how to clarify goals and priorities, the business of maintaining community groups, and how they relate to other groups and organisations and provide or run services. This way of dividing up the formation and functioning of community groups may seem arbitrary, but we have found it to be a useful means of covering and understanding a core part of neighbourhood work practice. Inevitably, we are aware of how our generalisations cannot apply to every category or type of community group. Their validity rests on the extent of our knowledge and experience of the field and on our judgement of their general applicability.

We explore the material in this chapter under the following headings:

from group to organisation;
forming an organisation;
building an organisation;
public meetings.

We attempt to identify the significant skill areas for the worker rather than to provide a comprehensive analysis of existing experiences.

From Group to Organisation

The emphasis given by Brager and Specht (1973) to understanding *organisation building* as a distinct phase seems to us to be a helpful way of developing an analysis of community group formation. Provided one is mindful that it will usually not be easy to separate this phase from other issues and problems a group will be facing, it is a distinction we suggest is observed. It forces workers to look closely at the components which together form part of community organising, rather than running them together either with the early formation of a group or with other issues an organisation faces once it has been formed.

It is a difference, essentially, between an informal group of individuals meeting tentatively to test out each other's interests,

commitment and general compatibility, and the deliberate formation of an organisation which has specified tasks to carry out and
which has some kind of constituency and legitimacy behind it.
While we continue to use the words community group within the
organisation phase, we shall maintain the conceptual distinction
between group and organisation, and hope to provide the reader
with a credible understanding of the differences between the two.

The substantial differences between a fledgling community group
and a group which has clear organisational characteristics often
receives only limited attention by both workers and groups. The
central question is: how will this grouping of individuals hold
together once they change from being an informal, often
temporary group to a more public and possibly permanent
organisation? Will the same people, for example, wish to
participate, or will the formation of an organisation require a
different set of capacities and skills from those used in a group?

The worker needs to help group members check out that they
do in fact share approximately the same understanding and
opinion about a problem or issue. It is essential for them to have
an awareness of what they are taking on when they shift from
being part of a group to an organisation. There has accumulated
sufficient experience in community organising for workers to
speak with confidence on this point: involvement of local people
over and above their other commitments can take a heavy toll on
domestic and social life. A neighbourhood worker who is working
closely with an active, busy group will be meeting one or more of
its members daily, while the members will be engaged in carrying
out a range of successive tasks. In addition, they will naturally be
drawn into informal discussion among themselves about the
group, and talk with neighbours, friends, relatives about their
work, often trying to encourage them to join in.

All this consumes time and energy of people who will often
have wives, husbands and families to support and who will face a
variety of economic pressures. Savill (1980), in a study of the
Association of London Housing Estates, records that some of its
leaders reckoned to spend about twenty hours a week on
association business. This may be unusually high, but the general
point about the implication of individuals committing themselves
to playing an active part in community organising, and the effects
of this on private lives, is applicable to most active community

groups. An understanding of some of the possible costs, as well as the benefits, of being involved in a group can be fostered by a neighbourhood worker as individuals move from being part of a loose, informal grouping to becoming members of an organisation.

Inevitably the process of forming a community group, and the tasks involved, will vary considerably according to local circumstances. Two important variables will be the extent of social interaction and community activity existing already in a neighbourhood, and the nature of the issue around which a group of people forms. The two variables are relevant whatever the predisposition of the worker may be, and we shall examine each in turn.

Community Conditions

What degrees of apathy exist in different kinds of neighbourhoods? What is meant by the word 'apathy' and how can apathy be recognised? These questions point to the severe problems facing a neighbourhood worker, both when local people appear to have little contact with each other, and when the worker knows very few people. This was the situation, for example, described by Popplestone in his study of collective action among tenants, and they at least rapidly found a common issue to bring them together:

> Action such as the formation of a 'successful' tenants association is more difficult to initiate than many realise. There were a huge number of unknowns, the significance of which needed to be taken into account. In the first place, the organisers knew few of the people in the neighbourhood. This made it difficult to know in advance who would most likely want to join. It also made it hard to know how to appeal to potential members. Doubly difficult in this case was the fact that neighbours in the area did not know each other and hence networks of communication had to be built up. (1972)

The first of four critical tasks suggested by Popplestone as means of strengthening a group is to provide a sufficiently enjoyable time when members come together for them to acquire a growing commitment as well as to accept the group's demands. The test is to enable the social benefits of joining a group to be carried over to the organisational phase of a group. Experience of neighbour-hood workers suggests that the need for social interaction in a group setting can be a springboard for effective community action in what has appeared to be a neighbourhood where very little is going on. Taylor *et al.* describe how workers can contribute to countering the effects on people of being labelled 'lazy', 'criminal', 'problem estates':

> It is possible to begin by involving people in such low-key community activities as playschemes for the children or simple social gatherings. Eventually, by a series of gradual steps, it may be possible to involve the community in such matters as negotiating planning decisions with authorities. (1976)

Participation in community affairs can challenge the negative stereotypes which outsiders hold of communities, and set in motion a positive cycle. The beginning of such changes is usually at a small and modest level where the activity strikes chords in enough individuals to make them want to come together, and to stay together as a collective unit.

A significant theme running through much community organis-ing during the last ten years is the extent to which neighbourhoods and groups of people who have been considered to be apathetic, unenterprising or depressed have demonstrated the vigour, initiative and skills which in fact exist in them. Neighbourhood work speaks to the strengths of communities. The willingness to be involved may need sparking, and this can be done as a result of a threat or a problem (rent increase, a main road planned to come through an estate, vandalism, etc.), through the energies of community leaders, or by the intervention of a neighbourhood worker; often it is a combination of all three. More recently, the experiences of working with unorganised or poorly organised groups of employees have driven home the same point: low-paid shift-workers, home-workers, night office-cleaners and other exploited groups have derived benefits of mutual support, as well as improvements in their conditions, through the efforts they have made to organise themselves. In doing so they have, at the same time, raised their own self-esteem and demonstrated their resourcefulness to others.

Neighbourhood workers, in contrast perhaps to the social scientist, are constantly looking for signs of interest and activity in communities which they can help to foster. By training and inclination they are motivated towards nosing out concerns in a community which are amenable to being debated and supported on a community basis. They are, in effect, in business to 'pick up' on issues which may be dormant in a community. This perspective may lead them to be relatively optimistic about the potential for action lying in so-called apathetic communities. George Smith and his colleagues explore this theme in their article on participation and the Community Development Project (1977) in which they are critical of academics who move too easily from the evidence of low levels of formal participation to the assumption that the poor are hard to organise. This they suggest, cannot be a tenable working hypothesis for a community worker:

> Rather than operate with a model of an apathetic community that must somehow be galvanised into action – or of a group which has calculated that it cannot afford the luxury of collective action, it is more appropriate to think in terms of a number of issues around which local groups are likely to mobilise, even if their response is not in a form likely to register on any formal index of participation.

Neighbourhood workers certainly need to become skilled at utilising existing informal networks of support and activity in neighbourhoods as well as capitalising on existing leadership. In the CDP literature it is pointed out that many of the projects were based in mining, docking or shipbuilding areas with a long history of collective industrial action, and that this made highly active community organising more likely to develop; it could be based on historical and existing patterns of contracts, networks and leadership. The fallacy is to transfer such conditions and activity to other communities seemingly facing similar problems. The process of understanding about a community and its history (as discussed in Chapter 3, Getting to know the Neighbourhood) has to precede the borrowing of tried organising strategies and tactics from elsewhere; it cannot be seen as an afterthought or as being of a secondary order to the business of working with community groups.

It would seem that there must be a tension between the neighbourhood worker's role as an agent of change, a facilitator, enabler and organiser, and the need to respect the existing fabric of the community where he or she works. It is one thing for the worker to have an adequate knowledge of the sociology of communities, it is another to apply it in practice to specific communities. Henderson (1978), in his appraisal of the Batley CDP, suggests that a major flaw in the project's strategy was the failure to accept in practice the implications of working in a close-knit, traditional community where the formal leadership patterns were extremely powerful; however energetic project workers were in encouraging informal and alternative leadership, they could not afford to underestimate the resilience and permeation of traditional leaders. There has to be awareness of different levels of community leadership as well as varying degrees of formality. How workers identify them, how and when they seek to get them interacting, remain questions which continually test their skill and judgement.

Community Issues

We turn now to our second variable influencing the transfer of an informal grouping of individuals to an organisation: the nature of the issue or concern which may bind them together and lead them to some kind of common commitment. The definition of an issue or starting-point for a group is well summarised by Baldock as 'the appreciation by people that they have a shared need or opportunity or problem' (1974). The seedbed for such a growth of awareness, and the length of time it takes for awareness to lead to organisation, naturally will depend on whether the issue arises out of debate within a small informal network, at one extreme, or out of a national or international social movement, at the other. These are polar extremes, and in between them there lies an infinite combination of possibilities, most of them involving at any one time national, regional and local factors.

Most issues around which people form are very localised and do not link directly to city-wide or national debates. The realisation, for example, in a community of the value of starting a good neighbourhood scheme for the elderly grows out of local people's own awareness of the need and what they can do about it. The influence of outside factors such as promotion by Age Concern or a policy statement by a government department, remain marginal.

Clearly related to whether an issue is predominantly local or national in origin is the question of the content of an issue. A high proportion of community organising in Britain since the mid-1960s has been around housing issues – clearance and redevelopment, rehabilitation and improvement, security of tenure, rent increases, maintenance and repairs, homelessness, housing co-operatives. The chances of forming a strong group when one of these issues is dominant in a community was relatively high. Play is another concern which yields high response in terms of community involvement, as witnessed by the rapid expansion of playgroups, playschemes and adventure playgrounds throughout the country.

If a worker is going to 'run with an issue', with the aim of gathering support as she does so, then she stands a good chance if it has to do with housing or play. Concerns which appear not to generate the same degree of immediate support might be a community arts project, the need for youth facilities and community care schemes for the elderly. Health issues may lie somewhere between the two: a hospital threatened with closure can mobilise community opposition rapidly; so too can health hazards to an entire community, such as that of the Carbon Black factory near Swansea in the early 1970s. Questions concerning the health of different groups of people have drawn increased interest and action more recently, especially around the idea of 'positive health' (Tetlow, 1979; Miller, 1979).

The above examples of the content of issues, and the broad divisions we have made, are generalisations. We underline their relevance, however, to neighbourhood workers who are in the position of judging when and with what expectatons they should assist with the formation of a community group. They can be helped in this critical area by drawing upon guidelines, based upon experience, both about the local–national focus of the issue or concern and about its content.

The worker can also make use of a more abstract framework. This can be portrayed as a scale which includes the decision of local people to form a group because they feel themselves to be under some threat, and the formation of a group because a number of people perceive an opportunity and decide to take it. It can be extended or made more sophisticated but may provide some guidance about the formation of groups (see Table 6.1).

In focusing upon the relevance of community conditions and

Table 6.1 *A framework for group formation*

Theme	Why Groups Form	Examples of Organising Issues
Threat	External threat	Major road planned through high-density housing area
	Intra-community threat	School closure
	Inter-communal tension	Asians and whites in London's East End
	Failing of power-holders	Inadequate repairs
	Response to an action perceived as unfair	Rent increases
	Accident to residents	Child falls from balcony
Opportunity	New resources	Community centre
	Significant change in composition of neighbourhood	Gentrification
	Change of political party in control of local authority	New policy on community centres
	Groups in other neighbourhoods are perceived to obtain success	Adventure playground

issues we have not attempted to answer the questions of why community groups do spring up. Rather, we have isolated two factors which influence the decision of a group to give itself an organisational form. Clearly there will be wide variation in the steps which groups of individuals take, and the length of time involved in each part of the organising process. It will depend, not least of all, on the kind of organisation which is being created: a youth project, a residents' association, a housing action group, a federation of tenants' associations will inevitably make different demands on people's organising capacities and need particular organisational arrangements.

Forming and building an organisation cannot follow any kind of blueprint. Yet it may be that a worker can offer invaluable help and advice to a group through her ability to separate out some of the relevant community conditions from the real or potential issues facing a group of individuals. When making contact, for example, on a Yorkshire council estate, a neighbourhood worker met people who formed part of a community where likely issues seemed to be camouflaged by habits and attitudes. The worker held a series of meetings with groups of women in their homes. The possibility of their turning themselves into an organisation to work on the need for recreational facilities – which they were identifying – did not advance. Nor was there a move to involve the male population in the discussions. Children's play, as well as forms of organising outside the workplace and clubs, was perceived as women's business.

Thus the nature of this particular community and the range of possible issues which could bring benefits to it were tightly bound together. It was the worker's task to be aware of this and to point out to those with whom he was working some of the difficulties they faced in this respect – when they were open to his advice, and when he judged he could offer his understanding of their community and the issues which could bring them together. Such general advice can complement work done on particular details of a group's formation. The importance of the worker judging when to intervene in this way will become clearer in the following section which analyses the range of possible tasks to be completed during the phase of helping the formation of a community group.

Forming an Organisation

The job of organising in the community can accommodate most kinds of worker style or character. Quiet determination, for example, can be as effective as extrovert charisma. The important 'mix' is between the personal qualities and strengths of a worker and his or her ability to maintain an awareness of the tasks which need to be undertaken – particularly as the organising becomes more hectic and demanding. We suggest that, rather than good organising been seen to derive almost entirely from 'secret' or natural talents, as much effort as possible should be given to making organising skills explicit. We propose to offer such an explication, first by setting out six points a worker can refer to when organising, and then by offering three general guidelines.

Checking Feasibility and Desirability

Neighbourhood workers rightly seek to remain close to their major brief: to help form groups. Their motivation and terms of employment focus on working with collectivities. Local people who are in contact with neighbourhood workers mostly have similar expectations. Yet forming a group is not necessarily or automatically always in the best interest of a particular collection of individuals. We have referred already to the internal strain group-organising can create on participants. Other factors to watch out for are the following:

Existing Groups   A group or organisation may already exist in the *same* area, and the worker may be confident that it can meet the needs of a group of individuals who are considering forming a new organisation. Why duplicate? The worker may often be in a position to advise, because people may be only semi-aware of an existing organisation, or not really believe one exists. This can happen on a large estate, especially when there is a high rate of mobility. Clearly the worker has to balance advice she gives about other relevant organisations with her understanding of some of the covert reasons why a group of people may want to start a new group (rivalry, personality conflict, status). She must also give due weight to one of the canons of community work theory: if people want to act together they have the right to do so, otherwise phrases about people expressing their own needs, unabetted and without interference, take on a hollow ring.

Neighbouring Groups   Equally, a similar organisation to the one being proposed may exist already in a *nearby* area. Would there be better pay-offs for both areas if interest and commitment within them were harnessed to one organisation? There could be benefits in keeping to one organisation which has sufficiently broad goals to encompass more than one set of interests; the common aims of each area might be achieved more swiftly and effectively. Examples could be found in housing areas facing similar problems or fighting for the same solutions; street groups could be more effective in one consolidated housing action group than if they each set up on their own, although this should not imply that workers should not organise on a street basis.

Potential Membership The likely membership of a proposed organisation may be small. If a neighbourhood worker, as a result of her experience and ability to analyse a situation, is convinced of this, why allow a group of people to move ahead under the illusion that active support will snowball? Failure, under these circumstances, would be inevitable and often destructive. If a worker thinks she can prevent this happening she need have no qualms about advising the group to hold back from starting an organisation. In case this appears to put too much power in the hands of the worker, we again emphasise the importance of leaving decisions in the end to those involved.

Timing It may not be an appropriate time for an informal group to move into an organisational phase. The members may not be strong enough as a collective; the situation around which they propose to organise may not be sufficiently clear; it may be important to wait upon the outcome of one or more external factors. There could be a number of reasons, in other words, why a worker might say in effect to a group, 'I am fully behind you, and I think you are doing right, but my advice is to wait a bit'.

Thinking About Strategy Finally, it is conceivable that the strategy of forming an organisation may in itself be a weak one, regardless of its timing. It may be, for example, that the last action a worker should encourage among young people on an estate where hostility to young people from adults is bitter would be the creation of a youth action group – not necessarily because of the worker's own values about escalation of conflict but in order not to worsen the lives of the young people themselves. Or, in an area of unemployment, it may be more relevant to concentrate energies on supporting existing organisations – trade unions and the trade council. Their first concern is with the place of work, but they could offer a base for taking action to deal with the effect of unemployment in the community, helping social security claims, for example, reducing boredom and frustration, or harnessing anger.

These two examples are given to emphasise the point that there need be no reverence for community groups as being good in themselves. Examining possible alternative or complementary approaches before making a commitment to organise can be a healthy means of checking on the feasibility and desirability of establishing community groups. It can also make for stronger organising.

Encouraging Leadership

Searching out and supporting individuals who can become leaders of community groups is of crucial importance in neighbourhood organising. For Alinsky,

> You talk to people through their leaders, and if you do not know the leaders you are in the same position as a person trying to telephone another party without knowing the telephone number. Knowing the identity of these natural leaders is knowing the telephone number of the people. Talking with these natural leaders is talking with the people. (1969)

Yet the identification of local leadership is usually a difficult task for a worker, and full of uncertainty. Much of his or her time will be spent in talking individually with those who have expressed an interest in taking on leadership roles – chairman, secretary, convenor, treasurer of a group, or simply being on the organising committee. She will wish to work through with each of them the duties involved when taking on a leadership position, what the commitment will imply in terms of time and energy, and how the assumptions of a leadership role will be viewed by other members of the group. At the same time, the worker will be trying to decide whether or not a particular person or persons will make effective leaders: Von Hoffman's warnings about plucking out 'natural leaders' have been referred to already (Chapter 5); wrong choices can mean early disaster for a group.

We shall see later that this element of uncertainty has implications for the early structuring of organisations. What, though, does the worker look for when wanting to encourage leadership within an emerging group? It is impossible to offer firm guidelines, or a checklist, of leadership qualities. It would, however, seem important that individuals can:

(1) demonstrate real *commitment* to the purpose of the group he or she will be involved with;
(2) *feel confident* that she can take on a leadership role;
(3) show she is aware of the need to hold the *trust and support* of the group, in situations which will sometimes test her stamina and loyalty;
(4) be committed to *democratic forms of organising* and to involving others.

These are just four relevant qualities for a leader of most types of community groups. The positive qualities which a potential community leader possesses can be the ones which cause difficulty later on – great forcefulness, strongly held convictions, for example. A worker will often greatly influence a group's choice of leaders by actions such as with whom she leaves messages or whose house she calls at. This may be held against her later. It is essential to continue to search out new leadership, and workers should avoid the temptation to go for 'safe' or existing leaders in the community when they are involved in helping to organise a group. Neighbourhood work tries to reach those without power, authority or status, sometimes groupings which are stigmatised by the rest of society. Leadership must come from within the groupings themselves.

More pragmatically, the choice or acceptance of a leader who already has some leadership role or status in the community can defeat the very purpose of organising, because people in a group will tend to feel that he or she cannot give a full commitment to it. Consequently their own investment in it will dwindle. In taking this view we do not wish to suggest that elected members, clergymen, youth leaders and others should never become leaders of community groups. We are offering, rather, a general principle for this key aspect of community organising against which a worker can compare particular practice situations. It offers a different focus from some writers on community work who imply that formal leaders must be involved in a community group from its inception. Ross, for example, states that:

Without the interest and support of these formal leaders, many difficulties would confront community organisation projects. Their participation is desirable because of their power, but also because they are able to communicate with individuals and groups in the formal social organisation. (1967)

We do not share Ross's conviction on this point, while recognising that in the real world there needs to be modification and sensible application of our general principle. It is certainly unwise, if not disingenuous, for workers to underestimate the amount of influence they can bring to bear on the process involved in choosing leaders.

Finally, we draw attention both to the amount of time to be put in by the worker when encouraging individuals to think about and decide upon taking up leadership positions, and to the value this can have for the individuals concerned. A worker is often welcomed into people's homes and talks at great length of hopes and fears for an emerging community group. At other times he or she will be involved in what may seem to be continuous hospitality in cafes and pubs, picking up key remarks made about forming an organisation and being introduced to new faces who could become future members of the group the worker is concerned with. She will aim to increase confidence of individuals at group meetings also.

The objective, in each instance, is for the worker to transmit her skills so that a group can take on increasing responsibilities and become more than a loose collection of like-minded people. Mitton and Morrison's description of Ilys Booker's role in the setting-up of the Nottingwood Playgroup Committee portrays well the gathering confidence of the group and of individuals' decisions to commit themselves and take on tasks and responsibilities:

It came about through raising funds. We had to have someone to look after the money, and everyone had to know what was coming in and what was going out, who was spending what money, and all this sort of thing. Before, I think Ilys looked after the money but Pat used to work out how it was spent, and then we decided, as the group was beginning to get going and was becoming self-supporting, that we would do it properly. It went very well. It was a new experience for all of us. I don't think any of us had done anything like this before. (1972)

179

The period between a decision in principle of a group of people to organise themselves properly, often represented by the setting-up of a steering committee, and the fruition of the decision, can be exhausting and depressing for group members. In addition, it not only provides opportunities for a worker to be extremely active, because of her knowledge and experience of how other groups have handled this situation, but it also requires her to be very open with group members as a person. The development of 'warm informal relationships' with individuals can make it easier for his or her advice to be acceptable. More important, it can begin to assure people of her willingness to go along with them. A related point about mutual support is made by Taylor *et al*. in the analysis of the worker's role at the beginning of the Waychester Project:

> It is also significant that a number of the group members looked on James as a personal friend, and that James also looked to them for support he did not get either from YVFF or from his local agency . . . 'I used to spend evening after evening with James when he was really down, he would come round to be brightened up. He was under a lot of mental strain.' (Mr Waters) (1976)

Our own and others' experience points, therefore, to the need for closeness and reciprocity between worker and group members, especially potential leaders, at this stage. The amount of time and energy involved in this kind of work, most of it outside any formal or public setting, is often underestimated by both workers and their employing agencies.

Early Help

We have deliberately separated the question of whether or not a worker takes a leadership role from the above discussion of leadership. Neighbourhood work seeks to encourage local leadership, it has as an implicit aim the devolution of existing sources of power – including that of the neighbourhood worker – in the belief that increased awareness and control by local people over a range of decisions has intrinsic value. *How* such a process is facilitated is another matter, but doubtless both directive and non-directive workers would agree on the above objective.

It may be that even the worker most committed to the non-directive approach may see it as both relevant and justifiable for him or her to assume some kind of leadership role in the formation phase of a community group. Leadership as a useful method of working with a group in the early stages of its formation can, in this sense, be distinguished from objectives and values concerning indigenous leadership.

Spergel states the case for a worker taking over the leadership role himself temporarily; there are times when he must 'step in and exercise clear and forceful leadership' (1969). Spergel is aware of the danger of this approach as far as a group and its potential leaders are concerned, and it is one we would give more attention to. Alinsky recounts a cautionary tale of how too much expertise and self-confidence by a worker can reinforce people's doubts about their own capacities and stop them from taking the first steps to organising. To themselves, the people of Muddy Flats thought:

> 'That smart New Yorker must certainly think I'm dumb – I've lived here for 40 years in all of this mess and that smart guy has to come around to tell me why I've been living in all this mess. What he's really saying when he tells me that I should come to that Friday night meeting is that I'm too dumb to know enough to do something about it. So if I go to the meeting I'm really admitting to him, and certainly to myself, that I am dumb.' So he doesn't go. (1969)

We are wary of introducing the notion of the worker becoming a leader – albeit a temporary one – of a group, or assuming a leadership role, because it puts so much on to the worker. Forming a community group does imply members taking some risks, and these cannot and should not be eliminated by the worker becoming a leader of the group. If she does, she is likely to store up problems for the group in the future, because she is placing them in a false cocoon. Sooner or later, when the worker may no longer be around, the group will become exposed and vulnerable to internal and external pressures, and it needs to be prepared for them. The worker should therefore resist temptations and pressures to take on a major leadership role which should be filled by a member of the group, despite the difficulties at times of doing so.

However, if the risks facing those who are forming a group cannot be eliminated, they can certainly be minimised by a neighbourhood worker. This suggests a different mode of leadership, and essentially takes the form of the worker offering services and help to the group, often in a direct and concrete way. They can be offered on a scale and with a degree of intensity at this point of the organising process so as to be able to contrast it with later phases, when help of the kind to which we are referring would certainly be misplaced. We suggest, in short, that there is value in a worker taking on a leadership role temporarily.

The most common form of early help provided by a worker is the carrying out of a plethora of small tasks. It could mean taking an active part in the planning and implementing of an initial fund-raising event for a group, such as a jumble sale: booking the hall, organising collection of items, obtaining and setting up tables, ensuring a rota of helpers, helping clear up afterwards. The worker's active participation in such tasks may have a twofold function: she may be showing people *how* to do certain things, such as booking a school hall through the local education authority and the head of the school, and she is demonstrating her own personal commitment to the group's future.

The notion of the worker showing he or she is prepared 'to get his hands dirty' revives mental images of Anglo-Saxon community development officers working alongside black farmers and labourers as they drive a roadway through a tropical forest. Yet despite connotations of condescension, the deliberate involvement of the worker in a group's early activities and her willingness to carry messages on its behalf is important and justified.

It goes without saying that the occasion and opportunity for this type of intervention by the worker will vary greatly. Some groups will have enough skill, knowledge, instinct and confidence to do without the worker; frequently they will be in the position of teaching her. Yet we suggest that many will not, and will benefit considerably from having the active help of a worker. For example, a playgroup committee which had been told it could purchase equipment at a discount from the education authority's store failed to act for several months. The worker involved was aware of the need for equipment reappearing, along with other matters, at successive meetings of the committee. It was only when he suggested he went with three of the committee, and involved himself in the enjoyment of selecting toys and games, that the necessary equipment was obtained, and the work of the committee progressed. Co-working between a worker and local leaders, whereby there are opportunities for learning and acquiring skills, can begin early on.

A variation of the above example is for the worker to inform a group which is organising about groups similar to itself and to suggest one or more visits. The groups might be at different stages of development, thereby enabling the visiting group members to have their ambitions and plans both re-affirmed and extended. The visits need not be limited to the area within which the group is located; for example, a group of people proposing to start a community transport scheme in Stepney went to Liverpool to see such a scheme in operation, in addition to visiting schemes in other parts of London. Naturally, the ability of a worker to offer this and other kinds of specific, task-focused help depends on her having sufficient basic knowledge of the availability of resources, and of how to find out about opportunities and resources quickly.

Awareness of the level and accessibility of resources required is perhaps the key to the ability of the worker to offer direct help, and to run errands for a group as it is in the process of becoming an organisation. It is a contribution which has been remarked on by several writers and confirmed by practitioners' experience. Goetschius states:

> Direct aid services are important early in the development of the group because the group has not yet found its own resources, and they are important to the worker in giving him something concrete to offer at a point when the group has not yet seen the full implications of his role or the scope of the service. (1969)

Anticipating

A more reflective task, which complements the sense of activity suggested by the provision of direct aid, has to do with the need to look ahead. What major problems or blockages is a group likely to meet and what should a worker do if she is confident of her forecast? Should she present her viewpoint to the group and thereby try to persuade it to change its approach, or should she leave it to continue, and possibly make damaging mistakes? Two brief examples will illustrate the dilemma we are pointing to.

(1) In a small mining town a community association has been formed on the initiative of an influential local doctor and two church leaders. Among its plans are the raising of funds for a community centre, the invitation of elected representatives to meet and discuss with its members, and the support of a junior youth club. The neighbourhood worker, while being positive about the association's plans, is aware that the organisation is dominated by a group of powerful individuals who are anxious to ensure their continuing control of all the association's activities. He feels this to be unhealthy as it merely confirms the existing leadership structure in the town and does nothing to alter people's feelings of powerlessness to act on their own. He starts to bring people together in one neighbourhood, chiefly around the issue of play, and immediately becomes aware of the association's concern to incorporate the groups within its structure.

   The worker thinks this would seriously weaken the groups, and tries to persuade them to resist the invitation and the polite but firm pressure of the association's officers. The groups fail to do so. They each retain a separate budget and committee, but within the overall structure of the association. In evaluating this piece of neighbourhood work, the worker considered he should have put his case to the groups much more strongly. He felt that their long-term effectiveness was diminished by being brought within the association.

(2) An unenthusiastic group of tenants in a block of flats starts to meet twice weekly and plans to form a tenants' association for the block. A neighbourhood worker is invited to the meetings, but feels there is limited scope for him to intervene: it is a group with too many ideas. Individuals put forward one after the other. Someone agrees to write them down but it is not made clear in what capacity he does so. The ideas range from projects (a cleaning rota for the lifts; outings for the elderly; a playscheme; a visit to the seaside), to fund-raising (a fete; a lottery; an art competition; a sponsored swim . . .) to political strategy (attending council committee meetings, requesting

officers of the local authority to attend public meetings; lobbying councillors . . .).

The stream of ideas sounds to the worker more appropriate for a strong, well-organised association which has gained some experience, rather than for a newly emerging group. He anticipates that few if any of the ideas will be put into action; individuals will become disillusioned and the early organisation of the tenants will break apart. Should he warn the group that this is likely to happen? How can he do this without blunting enthusiasm or appearing as a 'know-all' and risking moving the initiative from the group to himself?

These two examples illustrate not only how the worker has to engage in both 'technical' and 'interactional' tasks, but also the extent to which she has to anticipate the external as well as internal problems likely to befall a group. The first example demonstrates the need for workers to have a keen awareness of the ease with which an inexperienced group can be co-opted or sucked in by an existing organisation and thereby lose an important element of autonomy. We think the worker has a responsibility to alert a disorganised group to this possibility, and to spell out what the effects might be.

The second example illustrates how workers have to develop different group work skills in order to handle the various stages of a group's growth, in this instance how to warn the group of the likely consequences of its lack of internal control without dampening the all-important initial drive of a group. A worker's relationship with a group in this kind of situation, the skills she displays to them and the role she adopts, will contrast with her relationships once the group has formed. Many of them will focus on what Thomas describes as:

> acting as a clarifier of others' contributions, amplifying them, and translating them into other terms if they are misunderstood. Further he [the worker] might spell out some of the consequences of the various points put forward, leaving the meeting to decide what action should be taken. (1976)

'One thing leads to another'

Neighbourhood workers often carry in their minds the thought that out of the formation of one group will emerge others. There is nothing sinister about this. The awareness that new activities are likely to spring out of first initiatives reflects workers' knowledge of how and why people decide to join organisations and make them viable. If a worker were to misuse this knowledge, by abandoning or even sabotaging a group she had helped to form, or by unilaterally giving all her allegience to other groups in the locality, evidently this would be a form of manipulation and should be deplored. In our experience few workers act in this way. It would run counter to the strongly held value in neighbourhood work of encouraging a multiplicity of activities, of always encouraging systems to remain 'open'.

The awareness that small beginnings may lead to further community organising can be used by a worker helpfully and creatively. Generally, it can take two forms: a group may itself turn into either an extended or a different kind of organisation; or the formation of one group may stimulate the growth of others around related issues or common interests. In our experience, both of these patterns are likely to occur in neighbourhoods which are generally poorly resourced. When people see neighbours making progress on a particular issue, their confidence increases to a point where they decide to take action on other needs in the community.

Community Action has included several examples of the first form of one project leading to another. Often it begins with a small group of parents taking action over play. A report on play in London's Notting Hill by a local parent records how, over a period of six years, the number of playschemes and adventure playgrounds each multiplied about five times. Grants for community play projects increased also, and a fully staffed play association was formed to co-ordinate activities, with all of its staff local people.

The same report in *Community Action* also describes our second form of project development:

> In North Kensington organisations have come and gone like April showers and with the many saviours of the people. Yet community involvement in play is at its highest ever. Why is this? First these are the oldest and most consistent of all community activities and we can see on the ground the hard practical results of our efforts. But also once a group of parents

become active round a play site anything is possible: they start discussing other mutual problems – rent, holidays, food prices. This is the kind of thing that leads to advice centres, joint holiday plans, food co-ops etc. Some of the most active local people in the pioneering community projects in North Ken. started in play. (Smythe, 1973)

Workers of the Friends Neighbourhood House Project in Islington made use of a variety of play projects as a means of stimulating activity in neighbourhoods, and from these began helping the formation of tenants' associations in council flats scheduled for modernisation (Clarke and Henderson, 1978). This deliberate strategy evolved because the project had observed how play had led to many other schemes earlier on.

We have emphasised play in this discussion, but the notion of one thing leading to another can be applied to a range of activities. It may be particularly relevant to activities which people really enjoy doing: the 'fun element' in community work should never be underestimated. In addition to being valuable in itself, it can also lead to other forms of action. There is an important link here too between community art and neighbourhood work. We suggest that the notion of creative dynamic between one activity and others need not remain simply a haphazard possibility but may be thought about by the neighbourhood worker and shared with people she is working with.

Surveys

Neighbourhood workers frequently make use of surveys to assist community organising, and we have discussed them in Chapters 3 and 5. They can also be used alongside a number of other actions within an *integrated* strategy aimed at stimulating and encouraging organisation at a local level. The example by Foster (1975) of making contact on the Meadow-well Estate illustrates how surveys can form part of a strategy leading to organisation. The use of street representatives, and the holding of a public meeting, were essential ingredients of the use of the survey. It worked primarily as a community work intervention, and second, as an information-gathering instrument. Workers will be familiar with the experience of using a survey of the estate: they obtain a very poor response and very little information. Then the few people who showed interest come together. They re-word the questionnaire, organise the survey and collect useful information. That can be the beginning of a group.

Other techniques which can often be used in conjunction with a survey are video and a petition (ACW, 1979). The former can support a survey's findings with visual evidence and the voices of the people affected by a particular problem. The latter can be an effective means of capitalising on the results of a survey. People can be presented with hard information about their area or an issue and thereby be in a position to see the relevance of signing a petition. The wish to take action may be particularly strong if there has been a high involvement of local people in the survey.

The danger of raising too high expectations of action through use of the survey should be noted. It can lead to disillusionment about community organising. This points to the importance of clear thinking and detailed planning about how to make use of a survey as a means of forming a community organisation.

We have drawn attention to six categories of skill areas in the initial organising phase of neighbourhood work. There will be many others which workers draw upon; equally, those which we have highlighted will be applied in other phases of community groups too. Before we examine the tasks facing the worker when building an organisation, we shall end our discussion of the formation phase with three general comments.

Motivations of Group Members

First, a statement of the obvious: people give time and energy to community groups for a variety of private and public reasons. Motivations and aspirations of individuals inevitably influence the direction of an emerging group and the speed and ease with which it will become an organisation. People may first have to meet their own personal needs before they can solve the problems of others and of the community. Or such a stance may be rejected, and the thrust will be to help people make connections between their private ills and public problems. It is not within our brief to open this debate here. We wish merely to draw attention to the need for neighbourhood workers to remain aware of the degree to which motivations of group members are likely to differ, and for them to be able to respond to personal interests and demands within group or collective contexts.

An interesting set of arguments based on an analysis of why people do, or do not, decide to participate in collective action has been advanced by O'Brien (1975), making use of United States experience. His assumption is that people in poor areas have interests in common but that they are all self-interested individuals who try to be rational in coping wtih the problems of their lives. They may choose an individual solution rather than a neighbourhood organisation – often by fleeing the neighbourhood; O'Brien remarks that the greatest success in interesting people in neighbourhood organisation has occurred in minority-group neighbourhoods where discrimination makes the option of leaving less feasible. He suggests that the fundamental task of the neighbourhood organiser is to find incentives that will induce self-interested individuals to support collective efforts.

O'Brien touches on testing questions, in particular that of why poor neighbourhoods do not always organise spontaneously or easily. Such a rigorous approach to an understanding of those parts of practice which are often thought to be self-evident or unnecessary of examination has not yet been matched in the United Kingdom. It would require a careful analysis of why people do and do not become involved in community organising in different environments. The benefits for neighbourhood workers would lie in their increased ability to respond to the priorities and interests of local people.

The Wider Constituency

Evidence that a group of individuals is set upon forming itself into an organisation will draw a neighbourhood worker, who is in uncertain contact with it, into an initial working relationship. We have seen that the worker will wish to be identified with the efforts of group members, and that she will become involved in undertaking tasks for them. While she does these things she needs, as it were, to keep glancing over her shoulder at the wider community. Above all, she needs to retain the group's awareness of its wider constituency. In the example of the South Meadow-Well Residents' Working Group the organisers were careful to keep all tenants informed of what the street groups were doing and what the purpose of the survey was. A similar concern should inform action in an area divided between old-established residents and newcomers, where the latter are often scapegoated by the former for the area's deterioration. A continuing feedback process can be very important in these situations.

In its concern to organise itself, a community group can easily lose sight of the need and value of keeping in touch with neighbours who are not involved and with other local groups, both of whom may be affected by the group's subsequent action. Equally, in the situation where a group has come together with great difficulty and is very unsure of itself, it can be important for it to show the neighbourhood that it is alive and functioning by organising an event or activity early on – an outing for the elderly, a playscheme, even a duplicated progress report delivered to every household. None of these may fit the central purpose of the group, but by doing them the group may both help the necessary climate of opinion and retain its constituency. It will then be in a better position to continue and grow as an organisation. If the group concentrates solely on its own meetings – planning, discussing, developing – it will be perceived as inward-looking or as a paper organisation by others because there is nothing to convince them otherwise. In the long run, such early negative attitudes are likely to rebound on the group.

Clear Goals

Third, goals and objectives of a group which at the beginning seemed reasonably clear if not self-evident often start to appear complex, confused and elusive as time goes on. The worker has a vital role to play in helping a group to clarify its aims, and in ensuring that a period or mood of confusion does not continue. As new ideas emerge about how to tackle a particular issue, and as new members join the group, aims will naturally change. Again, the worker needs to be aware of shifts in attitude or position, of changes in aspiration and strategy, and work on them with the group. We shall see that this forms a key part of both building and maintaining an organisation.

The work at the early part, however, is equally important and may require the worker to be challenging, critical and provocative towards a group if she thinks its aims are unclear, woolly or overambitious. She needs, in effect, to be putting to the group the questions 'What are you in business for? What are you trying to do?'. Clarity and agreement on this will enable the group to work better on key questions such as membership, funds, timing and structures. *Community Action* lists the following as possible aims for a community group.

> To involve as many people as possible in a specific area in discussions of neighbourhood problems and collective action to meet them.
>
> To represent the interests of an area . . . and for it to be *seen* to be so.
>
> To bring together and represent the interests of a specific section of people.
>
> To fight on a specific issue.
>
> To run a project or service.
>
> To campaign on a broad issue affecting the whole borough or community. (1976)

It can be seen that the span of aims and objectives for groups is very broad. The worker should help a group be as precise as possible as to what it is trying to do before it moves too rapidly into an action-oriented and consolidating phase. By then there will be a number of other tasks to undertake, and it is well for them to be informed by a clarity of aims. The contribution of the worker on this point represents the keynote to the formation of effective community groups. Evidently there is a clear link with work done on clarifying goals and setting priorities once a group is established.

Building an Organisation

Ross (1967) echoes the feelings of many neighbourhood workers and community groups when he states that the reason why so many constitutions are formulated and then filed away and forgotten is that they do not represent a frame of reference for a group but rather a mechanical and meaningless ritual. Building community organisations, of which constitutions and operating procedures represent only a small part, calls upon the abilities of workers and leaders to make judgements about when to act, and what to introduce; every group will require a unique combination of organisational, professional, political and emotional support.

The period between the first early meetings of a group and the time when action begins to flow from the work and strength of the group is of paramount importance. There may be relatively little to show for it externally, yet it is the period when the foundations of an effective local organisation are laid. There will be many decisions to make and tasks to undertake. There will also need to be work done on the internal, interactional functioning of a group. We propose to exmaine these questions by concentrating on the following three areas:

(1) organisational structure;
(2) tactics and strategies;
(3) group cohesion.

Organisational Structure

The question of how organised a group should be continues to generate lively debate within community work. The authors of the Community Project Foundation's *Community Groups Handbook* report that 'the pros and cons of having a formal, organised group are almost endless and the people we interviewed had a wide range of views on the subject' (1977). It is a question, it should be remembered, which is relevant for all phases of the existence of a community group, because organisational requirements are likely to change as the nature and purpose of the group change. Cary has suggested that community organisations tend to develop through at least three stages: the initial stage of organisation, the task accomplishment stage and the stage of continuity or discontinuity. We are concerned at this point with the first of these. It is a time which places great demands on leaders: 'Persons with ideas and the ability to implement ideas contribute heavily during this initial stage' (1970).

Differences between kinds of community groups assume particular importance now. They increase the difficulty of generalising about organisational structure. The CPF's handbook identifies eight types of group.

Self-help groups: those which are run by the people who benefit

	from them, such as food co-operatives or mother and toddler groups
Welfare groups:	those which provide a service for other people, such as good neighbour schemes or advice centres
Representative groups:	elected by and answerable to the community – tenants' and residents' associations are obvious examples
Minority interest groups:	these are often self-help groups, but also try to improve the rights of certain sections of the population; examples are single mothers and black groups
Action groups: (or pressure groups)	these are self-appointed and take action in what they see to be the interests of the whole community; day nursery and anti-motorway campaigns are good examples
Liaison groups:	the authors regard these as only partly community groups, such as groups started by local authorities anxious to improve public participation between council tenants and a housing department
Traditional organisations:	well-established groups, usually catering for a particular sector of the community, such as women's institutes and working men's clubs
Social groups:	those which exist solely to put on social events; they range from loose groups of neighbours who organise an annual trip to Blackpool to quite large festival committees, sports leagues and associations for various hobbies (1977)

These are rough definitions of the different types of community group; many will fall into more than one category, and a further type could be added – that of 'ideological groups' (mainly political or religious) which are charaterised by having a philosophy by which they analyse a neighbourhood's problems and from which they find their strength. They may also be able to call on outside support for resources and for maintaining groups. Exmples range from church groups to socialists, environmentalists, pacifists, secret societies and political parties.

The typology helps us to appreciate how the organisational structure which is developed needs, above all, to be related to the functions it is going to play. Baldock (1974) argues that this factor is more important than that of the manner in which the group came together in determining the degree of formality or informality of structure.

We shall return to the question of formal and informal organisation after referring to three related issues which can be usefully differentiated in a discussion of the organisational structure of community groups.

Membership Most groups will start with a few people, and they will immediately be concerned with encouraging others to join them. The prior question, however, needs to be that posed by *Community Action* (1976) in its notes on membership: 'Why do you want members anyway?' The question is asked in order to encourage groups to be explicit about the advantages of having a large membership and to guide them in making effective use of members. It should not be assumed that membership is a good thing in itself. *Community Action* lists the following benefits: the more people involved in the group the more activities it can undertake; the more it can be aware of the issues that concern and interest people; the more it can be seen as representative; the stronger it is to undertake collective action. Greater fund-raising potential and a larger pool of skills and human resources to draw upon can be advantageous also. Yet there can be no firm guidelnes about the size of a group; too many members with no sense of real attachment to the group can be as damaging as too few.

As important as the number of members are the problems of staying in touch with existing members, and recruiting new ones. The first requires a two-pronged strategy: first, ensure that as many people as possible are involved at different levels of a group's activities:

> Not everyone has the same skills, nor can everyone devote the same amount of time to a group. A good example of this can be seen in the way a community newspaper is produced. The paper can be put together and kept going internally by a handful of people, but they will rely on a larger group to write articles for it, and an even larger group still to sell it. (CPF, 1977)

Second, make certain that there is good communication within the group: a regular newsletter if membership is large; reports of executive and other committee meetings. Such written methods can be complemented by encouraging verbal communication about the group. Each committee member, for example, can agree to pass on information to members of the group living close to him or her. Or personal contact can be maintained through weekly or monthly collection of subscriptions, but, in the words of *Community Action*, 'the collectors should make sure they leave time for the chat which can be as important as the money'. The vulnerability of community groups to loss of members and ultimately to failure is expressed convincingly in the same article:

> Perhaps the more common story of the failure of a group is the one where a group elects a small formal committee. The committee works extremely hard in the interests of the group, but fails to keep the wider membership informed and involved. The members feel that they aren't being consulted, that the committee is making all the decisions, and lose interest. The committee feel over-worked, unappreciated and finally give up, disillusioned with the 'apathy' of members. (1976)

Inevitably, groups will lose members, through waning of interest, other commitments or because they move from the area. One worker records how:

> Ever since I have been involved in tenants' associations on the estate, four years, there has been a continual drain because of committee members moving off the estate . . . Within a period of three months one particular committee lost through transfers two chairmen, the treasurer and a committee member. With such a steady depletion of the few that come forward to represent the estate one can see how extremely difficult it is to keep a committee together and to keep it active. (Palmer, 1978)

The natural process of loss of members, which contrasts with membership which declines because of misunderstanding or poor communication, will often give an edge to a group's desire to recruit new members. It is vital that a group has a continuing interest in this task, and it is as well for it to give one or more people the responsibility for ensuring the encouragement of new members. A group which has formed and is active can easily give the impression to outsiders of being exclusive, of not being interested in having new faces around. Such a situation not only runs counter to the search in community work for openness and avoidance of elitism but is also counter-productive to the group's long-term effectiveness.

Constitutions   Community groups usually benefit from having a written constitution. This simple statement leaves open the question of *when* a group should adopt a constitution; it is a question which is closely linked to the formal/informal organisation debate. Without a constitution a group lacks a tangible base point which says to the rest of the world: this group exists and therefore has a *prima facie* claim on the attention of others, as well as on other kinds of resources. Indeed, it is essential for groups to possess a constitution if they are to register with the Charities Commission, do fund-raising and if they wish to obtain rate relief. Without a constitution a group lays itself open to accusations of being a figment of activists' imaginations, or to expression of scorn and dismissal as irrelevant. It is foolish for a group to risk such attacks. A constitution can be viewed in these terms as a minimum organisational requirement.

In addition, the existence of a constitution can provide a strong backbone for the internal functioning of community groups. Not only is it there as a safety net if crises over leadership or policy arise, but it also legitimises the operating procedures of groups. These may develop intuitively with the formation of a group; the existence of a constitution will sanction them. In this way there is less likelihood of a group collapsing through confusion or disagreement over decision-making, the holding of elections or the accountability of committees or sub-parts of a group. Most medium-sized and large organisations will need to work a lot with a committee system. It is essential for the remit, responsibility and accountability of any committee to be clear, and the existence of a constitution can at least provide an agreed basis for reaching clarity.

Once again, different kinds of groups will require different constitutions. Some, like playgroups, community associations and citizens advice bureaux, meet few problems as they can draw upon model constitutions devised by their national bodies. Often, however, a suitable constitution will not be available for community groups, and a group will have to spend time on amending a constitution to meet its own requirements. Many tenants' associations in London, for example, make use of the constitution written by the London Tenants' Organisation in this way. This underlines the need for constitutions and rules to be seen as aids or enabling devices. Groups should use them as guidelines, not feel enslaved by them.

Premises The availability or otherwise of a meeting-place can have a profound effect on a community group as it struggles to become a strong organisation. We stress availability and access as opposed to ownership or tenancy. The latter, as will be seen in Chapter 9, raise different problems. Our concern here is to draw attention to the need for a group to have some certainty about where it can meet. This can apply at both an operational and psychological level.

It is a waste of a group's time and energy for it always to have to check out and negotiate the use of a room or building whenever it wants to meet. There will be many other things claiming the attention of organisers at this point and they should not have to worry about meeting premises as well. There is good sense in clearing away this particular hurdle at one go. Thus, if the group is a small one, agreement could be reached that meetings should rotate round each member's home (in such a case it is wise to warn against a process of competing hospitality as the group moves round; tea and biscuits one week can become sandwiches and cake the next, and can lead to unnecessary and distracting unease within the group!). For other groups, there is a need to establish a presence in particular premises – a tenants' hall, a local school, a church hall – so that there is a high expectation that it can use them again as it wants and not have to hunt around for alternatives.

Sometimes there will be overlap between premises used by a neighbourhood worker or community project and the meeting-place of a group. The combination of both in one set of premises would seem to offer potential benefits to both parties – workers and local groups. Yet ease of access to workers can place heavy pressures on them. This has been noted by Twelvetrees:

Apart from the strain on the workers it is impossible not to become over-involved at times as we are so near the situation. This makes it difficult for us always to look objectively at our work, which is vital if we are to be clear about what we are

197

trying to achieve, since the freedom and lack of structure make it easy for us to muddle on with no particular aims in mind, kidding ourselves that we are doing a good job just because we are busy. (1973)

One writer has described a variation on shared premises: a flat in the Gairbraid area of Glasgow was occupied by a fieldworker in order to provide a base for the project rather than as a resource for the community. Later, when made vacant, the flat became committee rooms and it, plus its telephone, proved to be indispensable for community organising in a situation of imminent housing demolition (Jacobs, 1976). A community group's need for premises will often change as it changes. Here, we have suggested that availability of a regular and agreed location can contribute to the early organisational development of groups.

Degrees of Formality Our discussion of constitutions has suggested what harm can be done when informally run groups come up against powerful, formal organisations. A group of London community leaders and workers noted that

> Some pensioners' groups are strongly against having a committee at all, since this divides the group and people more easily get left out. But problems arise – on both sides – when such groups have to do business with the formally constituted bodies set up by the local authority. (City Lit, 1978)

From a group's point of view, lack of a committee can mean there is no democratic control over those who want to set themselves up as leaders. Or it can mean that no one takes and develops special responsibility for the group: committees do not just have to be executive bodies. They and other forms of organisation can be set up to do specific tasks.

Brager and Specht make the point that the question of degree of formality poses another of the many community work dilemmas:

> On the one hand, informality is essential to permit expressive relationships to develop and for members to find satisfaction in the group. Conversely, however, if groups are to develop into institutional-relations organisations, rules have to be explicated, roles specified and other formal mechanisms evolved. (1973)

The neighbourhood worker has to help groups attain a balance between the need for informality and the development of formal structure. There will always be varieties of structures for groups of the same type, and the worker needs to remain aware of this when she makes suggestions to groups about how to organise. Baldock gives the example of a council estate tenants' organisation to illustrate this point. It might be:

> An organisation set up mainly to campaign over a particular issue run on a basis of frequent and regular decision-making public meetings with active roles (e.g. street organiser) given to a large number of members and a strong leadership core with charismatic features.

> An even more informal body based on a small area grouped around one or two individuals recognised as being competent by local people to speak for them.

> A highly routinised body with a strong federal structure in which there were a number of semi-autonomous sections for which the central committee acted as a co-ordinating mechanism.

> A body with a similar wide range of activities but with a stronger central committee and wider autonomy for sections making it easier to deploy all the resources of the organisation on a temporary (not necessarily political) campaign. (1974)

In striving to get the balance right for groups, the worker may be guided by the following consideratons.

(1) *How a group comes together* may help determine its structure. The group that forms around local informal networks should not ignore them when it decides upon its structure.

(2) Analysis of *the function of a group* can help to determine structure. Thus a single-issue or specialised group, like a playgroup, may be able to continue with a relatively informal structure compared with an organisation which seeks to speak for all the people in an area.

The organisational structures of housing co-operatives provide particularly important experience relevant to the above two points (which are both taken from Baldock, 1974); Anne Power (1977)

199

has written about the membership and management of co-operatives in North Islington.

(3) A clear danger is to advise a group to adopt formalised procedures too soon. They are then perceived as meaningless rituals. Members of a group will need *varying lengths of time* to respond to proposals for organising and the worker should be alert to indications that the group is moving too quickly for some members.

(4) It can be helpful for a worker to *estimate the pros and cons of proposed types of organisation* as openly as possible with a group. How far she can do this will depend on her relationship with a group and whether or not there are members who hold strong views on structure. These are often brought from other situations, such as the workplace or politics. How a group will be structured should reflect who the people are and how used they are to getting together.

(5) When a group decides to adopt more formal procedures, or conversely when it opts for an informal structure having used a formal one, *changes will occur in the group*. The worker needs to be aware of these and act if necessary. Thus a sensitive area, in the shift of a group from informal to formal organisation, will be that of leadership, because the power and influence of a chairman or secretary will become more explicit to members. Competition for leadership may accordingly increase. At the same time a worker can notice that a group which has been very anxious to establish formal procedures will often, once they have been obtained, neglect some of them and begin creating informal procedures. It is not, therefore, as if the move from informal to formal is a once-for-all matter. Rather it can be viewed as a continuum along which groups move unpredictably.

(6) Neighbourhood workers need to be aware of how *new approaches to organising in related fields* can be of direct relevance to their work. Two significant examples have been the women's movement and informal adult education projects. Workers can never afford to remain blinkered to developments which can inform their own approaches to helping groups establish appropriate organisational arrangements. Some groups, for example, have decided to let everyone who wants to have a go at being chairman, and then make a decision about whether or not a permanent chairman should be elected.

(7) Finally, *the position of minority or oppressed group members* should be considered. Many women, for example, seem to be reluctant to take on a chairing role, or are intimidated by formality, when they have much to contribute.

Tactics and Strategies

Increased confidence in the purpose of a community group, and a growth in commitment to it by its members, should be at the front of a neighbourhood worker's mind in building an organisation. Relevant organisational structure is necessary for any group. It is by no means sufficient. Indeed, on its own it will be arid. The essential accompaniment is the acquisition of organising experience by a group. Only with this kind of experience will people appreciate the extent of their shared need, opportunity or problem. It can take the form, on the one hand, of assigning roles and tasks to different members of a group. In this way, jobs which can include, for example, the production of posters, distribution of a newsletter, and establishing links with local newspapers, together form part of a process whereby a strong group identity is created.

The other form of organising experience builds on the idea of collective activity, in contrast to the tasks referred to above which can seem more individualistic even though they are being undertaken on behalf of a group. A worker's encouragement of a group to act with a collective purpose should focus on two areas, the strategic and the tactical.

Strategy is concerned wth the long term, and it implies consciously planned action based, as far as possible, on an understanding of cause and effect of a particular state of affairs. It assumes a rudimentary analysis of power and it presupposes political knowledge of the influence and the strengths and weaknesses of relevant individuals and organisations. Tactics are best conceived as methods of action, using resources to attain goals or objectives. They are to do with anticipating the moves of others, and with the consequent detailed planning and manoeuvring.

A range of tactics does not add up to a strategy. Tactics are the equivalent of a planned series of battles, not a war. A war presupposes broad, underpinning strategies on the part of contestants. Yet tactics are more than skirmishes. They should be considered moves which relate to each other in a loose logical way. A community project may adopt a strategy of working towards better local understanding of the housing market; the tactics it deploys could include research into local authority allocation policies, supporting housing groups and analysing tenure patterns.

A community group may aim to achieve better housing and recreational facilities in an area by securing increased participation of local people in decision-making processes which affect the area. This can be classed as a strategy. It will engage, however, in successive clusters of tactical actions. It will also, if it is wise, set less ambitious targets and achieve them before setting new ones. Finally, it will prepare itself on a number of fronts: collection of information, formulation of arguments, finding out where best to present arguments and how, establishment of an internal system for keeping copies of correspondence, and so on.

All these activities will demonstrate that a group is thinking in tactical as well as strategic terms. Alongside them will occur specific pieces of action: organising a petition, leafleting an area, a demonstration, fund-raising events. By themselves, each one of these actions would have minimal impact. They need to be seen by members of the group concerned to relate to each other, to contain their own dynamic movement towards a particular target or objectives. Notes in *Community Action* on organising a petition capture well the importance of interlocking pieces of action:

> Remember that a petition is just one weapon, and in most cases, a relatively minor one. You must decide whether a petition can be used as part of your overall plan of campaign. A petition is, in effect one part of the reasoned argument of our case. (1975b)

Only when the possible advantages of a petition have been fully investigated, and tested against a group's overall strategy, should the remaining questions be tackled: deciding how to use a petition, the form of a petition, and organising the collection of signatures.

Introducing the distinction between strategy and tactics at this point in our discussion of the formation and building of community groups is done for two reasons. Firstly, there is a tendency for groups to organise on a 'crisis' basis. They respond to given situations – pressures, threats, opportunities. After a time, if they have not begun to form clear ideas about what they want to do and how they should do it, this becomes a very weakening and demoralising position. That theme in community work which encourages open participation, flexible non-bureaucratic structures and spontaneity needs to be counterbalanced by working with groups on the need for thinking at both strategic and tactical levels. Otherwise they will never be masters of a situation. They will always be on the run. Countering such a tendency implies putting to a group the principles that the basis of action should not be a moral one alone, that feelings about a particular target can usefully be separated from cognitive tactical judgements.

The second reason for suggesting consideration of strategies and tactics at an early stage of the organising process relates to the importance of preparing a group. Groups will have to make decisions about policy and action once they are heavily involved in issues, and they can best do this as a result of being familiar in their thinking and approach with the distinction we have made. A major task of neighbourhood workers is to help groups represent their interests to other parties effectively, and to make use of opportunities when they arise. Encouraging groups to think in strategic and tactical terms from the time that they decide to become an organisation can result in long-term benefits. There is an excellent discussion of strategies and tactics in community work in the book by Brager and Specht (1973, pt IV). The work of preparing a group for the future can be helped in at least three ways.

Practising   A group can be encouraged to practise skills, either by rehearsing a proposed action or by agreeing to analyse and criticise the performances of group members rigorously and openly. It could decide, in other words, to put time aside in the early period to practise and learn through doing. The support and involvement of those in leadership positions and of the neighbourhood worker involved could be crucial to such an exercise. It lends itself also to the use of video.

Members could discuss a likely scenario: a first meeting with the local social work team, an interview with a trust to support an application for funds, door-knocking to recruit new members. They could role play these imaginary situations, watch the video recording and pick out the weaknesses; they could then do the role play a second time, and be aware of improved confidence and the application of explicit skills. This use of video is similar to the way trainers use it in workshops on neighbourhood work skills. It is remarkable how many obviously weak areas can be corrected by this method; the failure, for example, of someone to introduce himself properly at a first meeting, or the domination of an encounter by a minority of those present. Practising and rehearsing in this way can be equally useful for community groups.

Clarifying the Worker's Role We have emphasised already the need for workers to make their role and relationship with the groups as clear as possible. Often at the early stage of a group's formation this will be difficult, and should not be insisted upon. However, as a group gains strength, from a sense of solidarity as well as from getting itself organised, the need for workers to clarify their role, and what they can do for the group, becomes more relevant. This can be particularly important if a worker is both an enabler and a member of a group; she is holding more than one role. A mental health group or a women's group would be good examples.

Workers can stimulate an awareness of their role by sometimes taking on almost a participant observer role with the group. Such a capacity to be detached from the group while at the same time being trusted and needed by it can be helpful to a group and not interpreted as undermining its collective identity.

Setting Targets Finally, a group's preparation can return to the matter of setting realistic objectives and understanding the target: it is no use battering the estate manager if the decision has to be taken by the housing committee. A careful and anticipatory discussion of what a group can hope to achieve within an approximate time period can be salutary, and result in some reformulating or modification of early objectives. This can be of lasting value.

A group is likely to survive and be effective if its members know that each of them will carry through the responsibilities they have agreed to undertake. A testing-out process, whereby expectations on individual members and the group as a whole are assessed, can be an essential part of the growth of any group's political literacy. Such a familiarity with political processes has to include how a group manages its affairs, how control is exercised, how decisions are made and how responsibilities are allocated.

Group Cohesion

Neighbourhood workers tend to talk enthusiastically about their work; those who do not will generally move on. In catching and conveying the excitement of community organising, however, they may unconsciously sidestep some of the major blockages and frustrations experienced by a group once it has decided to organise. The pattern, in reality, of the development of most groups is uneven. There may be a lengthy period while a group awaits a reply from the local authority about resources or a meeting. It is in situations like these that the neighbourhood worker has to work hard to keep a group together. Although it may be intent upon achieving its organisational goals, it will remain vulnerable to unexpected buffets, changes of plan, personality conflicts or struggles for leadership.

Here we focus briefly on the tasks of workers in looking after the internal processes of a group, compared with 'external' tasks such as broadening a group's constituency and building 'outside' support or coalitions for a group. The latter tend to form a more central part of the organising process. We have referred to them earlier in this chapter and they retain a major importance throughout the neighbourhood work process – to a greater extent perhaps than the need for internal work at the organisation-building stage. The aim of any internal work done with a group will be to ensure its continuing cohesion and to encourage further growth of felt unity and collective purpose. Some of the forms it can take are as follows:

(1) *Countering depression within a group about apparent lack of progress or unanticipated obstacles* – consistently low turn-outs at meetings organised by the group, for example, or failure to obtain an early inflow of funds for the group, or unexpected opposition from another group of local people, or simply an entrenched and demoralising feeling that whatever the group does it will have no significant effect, an experience conveyed by Palmer:

All around them in their daily lives tenants see examples of retrogression and conclude 'that things are getting worse'. One of the problems at committee meetings is to persuade people to plod on even though there appears no reason at all why they should. A number give up through sheer frustration at the difficulty of the job, and who can blame them?

So, committees can slowly crumble, if not through key members leaving the estate, then because of members' own inexperience or frustration at the difficulty of the job. (1978)

Somehow the worker has to find ways of trying to help a group move away from a feeling of being 'down' in this way. She can refer to the achievements of groups in other similar areas. She can point to evidence of a group's work which justifies hopefulness rather than despair. She can suggest new activities and introduce discussion of different tactics. Clearly, however, she will not be armed with instant panaceas. Often it will be a matter of helping hold a group together until it rediscovers its sense of purpose by itself.

(2) *Working with leaders individually.* Every neighbourhood worker will have a preferred style of operation. Some workers, for example, will keep formal meetings and documentation to a minimum and utilise a range of informal skills, while others will prefer the reverse. This is partly a question of individual preference or predisposition and partly a value question about how directive a worker decides to be. Most workers, however, see the need to work closely with the leadership of a group in its early days, with a lot of emphasis being placed on bolstering the confidence of leaders. This can best be done individually, and much of the time of a worker can be spent in informal discussion with a chairman or secretary in his or her home. It represents the private, face-to-face dimension of neighbourhood work in contrast to the more familiar public nature of the work.

It is important for that kind of support not to be limited to designated leaders of a group but to include others who play leading roles – the ideas person, for example, or the practical person. The worker can help to ensure that there are more than one or two leaders in a group, and thereby prevent it from becoming dominated by a small clique. As well as providing support in this way to individual members, the worker can also share her concerns about the group. These can include the need to expand the leadership of the group, despite the problems this sometimes poses. Cary (1970) notes that the initial stage of organisation involves fewer participants than other stages.

It is also essential to try to avoid leadership or the initial nucleus of a group from becoming skewed in favour of the higher status or socio-economic groupings within a community. There is abundant evidence to show that participation is not uniformly distributed throughout a community. If a worker thinks that a minority section or a significant part of the community is not represented in the group, she should share her anxiety openly with the leadership. It will usually be easier, and more productive, to do this early on in the life of a group, when there may exist more flexibility and openness, rather than leave it for later.

(3) *Assessing the pace of activity by a group.* A worker's frequent contact with the leaders of a group needs to be complemented by a critical view of the pace being set for the group as a whole. Is it appropriate to the aims and objectives of the group? Is it too fast or too slow for the total group, as opposed to a majority or minority within it? A worker who is part of a community work team is at an advantage when doing this kind of assessment because she can check it with colleagues. The study of a youth and community work project in East London by John Edginton (1979) includes very useful discussion of team work.

A worker has to be prepared to give her views to a group she is supporting, even if this may cause some irritation within the group. She may feel, for example, that the plans and programmes of a group are advancing too far ahead of the process of acquiring particular skills among members, and she would argue for time being spent on developing them – chairing a meeting, public speaking, keeping accounts. We continue discussion of the worker's role in furthering the development of a group in Chapter 8.

Public Meetings

In Chapter 5 we discussed the public meeting as a way of initially contacting people. We return to public meetings here in order to indicate some of their other functions. Such a discussion is particularly opportune because it may correct any impression conveyed of a clear dividing-line between the work of forming an organisation and that of building it. In practice situations the two run together. We have used the distinction, in the same way that a neighbourhood worker might use it when reflecting upon her practice, in order to draw attention to particular tasks and skills within the formation and building stages. Examining the topic of public meetings, which are frequently the focus of community organising, may help to draw together the themes of forming and building and to demonstrate the major characteristics of the worker's role.

The decision of a group to hold a public meeting is frequently its first major endeavour to test the interest and support of its wider constituency. Implicit in the decision will usually be a desire both to confirm the work of the organising group and to draw in more members. 'Meetings should build the oganization and lead to action' (Norton, 1977). In such situations, a fledgling group is investing and risking a lot in a public meeting, and it is vital that the group gets it right. The key to this may lie in the extent of a group's awareness that the public meeting is *its* meeting. *Community Action* emphasises this point in order to avoid invited councillors or outsiders taking over a meeting: 'If you do invite them, work out your questions for them well in advance. *Don't* let them share the platform at large public meetings – it's *your* meeting.' (1974)

Such advice is fair, and points to the need, first, for a group to see a public meeting as part of an organising strategy and not as an isolated event. Second, it underlines the need for clarity about the purpose of a meeting. *Community Action* has listed the following likely purposes of a public meeting:

(1) To find out what people in the area feel are key issues.
(2) To raise issues, get approval of demands and ideas for action.
(3) To use the meeting to form a tenants' association or action group.
(4) To build up and strengthen an existing group and make it more representative.
(5) To launch a campaign, get publicity for the issue, etc.
(6) To explain and discuss the progress of a campaign and to get support for further action.

(7) To show that your demands and proposals have wide support and to use this to show that the group is a force to be reckoned with.

(8) To get representatives from the council, other public bodies, organisations, or firms to listen to residents' demands and explain what they will do about them.

(9) Hold the association's or group's annual general meeting. (1975a)

The purpose of a public meeting could be one or more of the above. A group needs to work on the issue of 'why hold a meeting?' in relation to its other activities and plans. Then, when it moves ahead with organising the meeting, it can retain some control over it by drawing upon the strategic and tactical thinking we have suggested a group needs to engage in from the beginning. The Table 6.2 illustrates some of the opportunities available to a group when it is entirely responsible for organising a meeting, and contrasts it with the situation of a group entering a meeting where it has little idea of what to expect.

Planning and management of public meetings calls for skilful judgement by a neighbourhood worker as well as by community groups. In a sense, issues around a public meeting epitomise the demands made upon two main skill areas throughout the forming

Table 6.2   *Preparing for a public meeting*

	Strategies	Tactics
Known situation	Why have it? Who should be there? What do we want from it? Who will organise what?	Leaflets and posters Newsletter Rehearsal Seating arrangement Prepared questions Priming the press
Unknown situation	Who will be there? What are we all agreed on? What kind of meeting is it – exchange of opinions or negotiating?	Clarify purpose Suggest seating alteration Adjournment Spokesperson Note-taker

and building process: an excellent *sense of timing* – when to introduce specific ideas and techniques to an evolving group; and an ability to *think strategically* and to be able to convey such an approach to community groups.

Both skills retain their importance throughout the organising process, but they first attain major significance at this stage. Both, it should be said, sometimes appear to be handled by workers and groups intuitively or by hunch: a worker, for example, who had been involved with a small group of tenants for more than a year and who had been unable to link it with a young group he was also working with on the same estate decided to attend what he thought would be another inconclusive meeting. To his surprise, membership had revived, and during the meeting sufficiently positive comments were made about the value of the youth activities being organised for him to suggest that the two groups should get together in order to improve facilities on the estate. The group agreed to it. The worker could think of no rational explanation for this development. Like a lot of neighbourhood work, it was a combination of the place, the time and the people.

We are aware of the danger of implying that every group will move, with varying degrees of difficulty, through the formation and building phases. Clearly they will not. Many informal groups will fail to become organisations. It is impossible to predict with certainty the passage of community groups because they must retain their autonomy, and because no human activity, least of all neighbourhood work, can be programmed to unfurl tidy and controlled plans and actions.

CHAPTER 7

Helping to Clarify Goals and Priorities

Clarifying Goals
Identifying Priorities
  Nominal groups
  Delphi

Issues for the Worker
  Role
  Framework for action
  Constraints on workers
  Recording
  Standing back

The need for community groups to clarify goals and identify priorities is integral to the forming and building of organisations discussed in the last chapter. They are necessarily linked to strategy formation. Clarification of goals and the identification of priorities are also closely connected with each other.

It is important to give attention to the question of how groups consciously work through the process of deciding upon goals and priorities. It is also imperative to focus on some key implications for the neighbourhood worker when a group is organised to the point of acquiring experience and gaining confidence about what it wants to achieve. We shall explore these two themes by discussing in turn the need for community groups to examine goals and set priorities. We shall then identify some issues for workers.

We preface our contribution to this area by noting that the requirement for rational thought needs to be considered within an analysis of class and community work. How meaningful will a worker's attempt be to introduce issues of choice and decision-making, based on explicit criteria, with working-class groups? There will be ability to grapple with the issues, but initially there may be a lack of familiarity with them. A worker may be able to show the similarity of group members' other activities at work

211

and in the community, such as trade unions, sports and running a household; in these activities people regularly set goals and priorities without describing it as such. This point relates to Tasker's discussion of the central role of administration in the lives of working-class people, and of how at the workplace 'the working life of manually employed people consists of being in the situation of receiving instructions to an almost total extent' (1978). It is clear to us that explicit discussion of goals and priorities will be among the more difficult tasks for community groups. Accordingly a worker needs to approach this area with sensitivity, and be prepared to adapt considerably her plans for tackling issues of choice.

Clarifying Goals

There are dangers of reifying the search for clear goals. They can come to seem highly abstract. Using the distinction between goals and objectives may exacerbate the dangers, yet it is a valuable distinction and one which we adopt. Goals are the highest level of objectives. They lack specificity, they stand out as statements of value and they are not easily attainable. Objectives, on the other hand, are concerned with specifics, they suggest what action is implied and what targets should be attained. They relate directly to strategies and tactics. This use of the term 'objectives' has the effect of reinforcing the abstract connotation of 'goals'.

Most organisations have multiple goals rather than a single goal, and this is as true of small, newly formed community groups as it is of established organisations. Multiple goals do not necessarily imply confusion or contradiction within an organisation. Astin describes three functions of the emergent Oxford Rights and Information Forum:

> firstly, as a general co-ordinating and information sharing body; secondly as a training resource in the field of welfare rights . . . and thirdly, as a pressure group in the field of welfare rights. (1979)

In addition, organisations' goals are not static, they shift over time. Rothman (1969) suggests that it may be useful to view an organisation's goals from a historical perspective. Either one goal is substituted for another ('goal displacement') or new goals are added when old ones have been achieved or cannot be obtained ('goal succession'). From the viewpoint of the sponsors, several of the Community Development Projects substantially changed their goals over a period of five years; few sponsors could have anticipated the ideas put forward by CPD in later publications which advocated explicit political programmes. Early documentation perceived the project chiefly in terms of improved local and national co-ordination.

Goal development is an ongoing process which is 'all the more complicated by the fact that there are three actors (i.e. constituents, workers and sponsors) attempting to influence the outcome'. Brager and Specht also suggest three ways in which organisations can deal with differences among goals:

(1) When the objectives are viewed by participants as compatible, compromise is possible, and two goals may be sought at once; (2) a second form of compromise is accomplished by 'planned ambiguity', a form of adjustment which occurs when a group's objectives seem to conflict; (3) the third method is to achieve clarity by choooosing one goal as primary from among conflicting claims, discarding others, or assigning them a lower priority. (1973)

The example they provide for the first form of compromise, the welfare rights movement, is as appropriate to the British context as to the United States: those in leadership positions frequently see the mobilisation of claimants as a means of bringing about change in the income maintenance system; but claimants are often intent on achieving more modest and short-range ends, such as an increase in emergency payments. There is evidence to suggest the feasibility of retaining both goals at the same time. However, the difficulties of doing so should not be underestimated.

The idea of planned ambiguity of goals is given considerable significance by Brager and Specht because ambiguity is 'more advantageous to the *least* powerful members of the coalition': the clearer the goals, the more influential become existing leaders of a group or organisation, 'in effect, the precise goals of organisations represent the clarity of their most powerful members'. The advantages of planned goal ambiguity will clearly make considerable demands on the worker's skills.

Within community work literature, Rothman (1969) has shown how specific objectives are inherent in community work practice, but they exist alongside less tangible 'process goals'. The latter refer – in simple terms – to educational aims whereby local people, through their experience of organising together, develop and change as individuals and groups. They are broad goals which are focused on 'growth' or 'maturity' in civic affairs rather than on the solution of a particular problem or the meeting of a special need. We have seen how it is associated in particular with the work of Ross, W. and E. Biddle and Batten. It has been taken up both by those concerned to evolve new forms of adult education and by followers of 'consciousness-raising' methods articulated by Freire. It contrasts with the achievement by community groups of specific tasks. Rothman suggests that the use of the terms 'process' and 'task' goals causes confusion, partly because process goals often contain concrete tasks. Our purpose here is not to pursue this conceptual argument but to emphasise the tension which often faces a community group between sustaining its own cohesion and fixing on a clear set of goals and objectives.

In what ways can there exist tension or competing claims between the internal functioning of a community group and the clarification of goals and objectives? In earlier chapters we have referred to the importance of a group developing a collective identity, and how this can often begin through social relationships and informal interchanges which help to bind people to a group. As a group turns towards working out in specific terms what it intends to achieve the 'togetherness' and unity of the group may be put under strain. Basically this happens because differences of view about the group's goals emerge. There are at least four ways in which this can happen.

(1) *Pressures on members.* Strong personal disagreements may be exposed, which often are inseparable from conflicts of personalities. This can occur once the effects of a group's activities begin to be recognised in the community or by agencies, and the group thereby experiences both positive and negative pressures. The message is driven home that being a member of a group can have serious implications for the individual. It is one thing, for example, when a group announces it is to open an advice and information centre, but those involved will face a quite different kind of reality when they undertake their first supplementary

benefits tribunal case or challenge the local authority's housing policy by a demonstration. It is then that those most committed to the advocacy role of the centre will be perceived by other members as 'the most powerful individuals'. They will accordingly be able to place their stamp on the group's functioning, because they become the leaders in a situation of covert disagreement among the membership or constituency about the group's goals.

(2) *Formal and informal priorities*. It is quite possible for a group to retain its 'celebratory' element, the socialising, the fun and enjoyment which form such a vital part of community organising, with the furthering of more serious activities. Indeed, both a neighbourhood worker and a group's leaders will usually strive to ensure that these do not become lost as the group increases its 'work' activity.

In his description of the formation of Gosford Green Residents' Association, Benington (1975) notes how the spirit of the meeting was one of excitement and that the forming of the committee at the end was done 'fairly informally, people in the hall suggesting the names of friends and others they knew in the area'. At the same meeting it was agreed what the committee's first steps should be and that there should be frequent public meetings to report back progress and discuss developments. In this instance, therefore, there was a close connection between the informal and the formal elements of organising.

Inevitably, however, some members will feel less committed to furthering a group's main aims than others. The important point is for the group not to allow that natural division or sets of preferences to divide it. Those people who are seen to do the 'small tasks' — social secretary, delivering envelopes, locking up — or who cannot give as much time to the group's work as others need to receive recognition of their contributions by those who set the pace of the group in terms of its main work. Otherwise the group will lose them, and be so much the weaker.

(3) *Conflicts of interest*. There will often be clear-cut conflicts of interest within a group which are only revealed as its goals become clarified. Such conflict may turn upon differences of viewpoint, values, ideology between individuals about proposed policies and actions, or it may emerge as the issue or content area with which the group is concerned is better understood. An example might be plans for a motorway to go through an area; if

215

an individual is only going to be minimally affected by it he or she is less likely to stay an active member of a group campaigning to stop it. In neighbourhood work it is essential for a worker and a group to be able to judge when certain goals have or have not been achieved. In the latter case, if conflicts of interest become counter-productive or 'planned ambiguity' loses its validity, it may become necessary for a worker to help a group stop meeting.

(4) *Ends and means.* It is artificial to study goals without relating them to the means or methods by which they are to be attained, or without recognising that the two interact. *How* you are going to achieve something can be as important for some people, in terms of their involvement, as what it is proposed to achieve. Some people, for example, will support a housing association which aims to extend housing availability but will relinquish that support if the association becomes involved in squatting. In that case there can be no disagreement about goals, but considerable divergence about how to achieve them. We shall see in Chapter 9 how there can be fundamental differences between a group's decision to provide a service and a decision to campaign, and how they may each rely upon different individuals to support them.

Management specialists have developed a number of formats and step-by-step guidelines for goal and objectives setting. These can be used to ensure that actions both derive from and contribute to social and individual values. One approach which may be of particular use to neighbourhood workers is that called the 'key results' exercise, because it can be undertaken by individuals and small groups. Its methodology is that of the management by objectives approach, and it is essentially a method of relating the targets and objectives of the individual to the goals of an organisation to enable the one to help determine the other. It allows individuals and small groups to be clearer in their work, to have a strong measure of self-control, to make explicit their activities and to be self-regulating and self-appraising.

The 'key results' exercise is set out below as a very simple planning schema. It should be changed around to suit the particular circumstances of groups.

(1) *Goals/objectives.* What overall improvements do you personally want to see achieved in the next year? Make sure that

you are talking about effects to be achieved rather than activities.

(2) *Evaluative criteria.* How will you know you have achieved any of the goals or objectives – marginally, substantially or completely?

(3) *Action.* What activities do you need to undertake to achieve your goals/objectives?

(4) *Blockages.* Who or what will prevent your achievement of goals/objectives? What will you do to counteract these blockages?

Neighbourhood workers may find the material emanating from management training too restrictive or find its terminology off-putting. The case for community workers to make use of planning and management studies to help them develop systematic approaches and methods for handling problems is discussed by Algie, Miller and Kam (1977). They can be relevant to a worker's own planning as well as that of groups.

Before we discuss the question of the identifiation of a group's priorities it is important to emphasise the crucial part that goal clarification plays in the neighbourhood work process. It is, first, an essential link between a worker finding out about a community and the development of a strategy and programme which will be relevant to that community. The groups he or she comes to work with need to be aware of that connection. Their growth cannot be divorced from the actions and thinking of the worker.

Failure to think through the goals of a group is frequently the weakest point in a group's life and in the organising process. It is when confusion, frustration or failure is most likely to happen. Once again, we see the need for choices about a group's direction to be basically strategic ones. An approach should be selected with a view to achieving specified goals and objectives, not just in order to proclaim a statement.

Second, spending time and energy on a group's goals is essential if the idea of evaluation is to retain validity. Without clarity about goals, there will be nothing against which to measure the achievements which may be claimed. As a result, the continuing sense of movement of the process idea becomes lost. It comes to be a once-and-for-all device rather than a flexible, cyclical one, and considerably less useful as a result. We discuss evaluation in Chapter 9.

Identifying Priorities

For an annual meeting of the Association of Community Workers one contributor wrote:

> Community work is . . . becoming increasingly characterised by its need to order priorities in developing its work programme, primarily because of its limited resources, staff, finance and time. In ordering these priorities community workers are likely to be governed by at least two criteria. Firstly, that of the nature of local problems and the degree to which they make impact on the community. And secondly, but possibly less obviously, the possibilities of attaining some success, however that may be defined, in any particular area of activity. (Spence, 1978)

The usefulness of this statement lies in the emphasis placed upon the need to base choice of priorities upon criteria, rather than (for example) upon impulse or upon 'what seems best'. This applies as much to community groups, especially in the early phase of their formation, as to neighbourhood workers. By criteria one means, in this context, agreed and articulated reasons why a group chooses to concentrate upon one issue or project rather than another; a group proceeds, for example, with organising children's playschemes because it thinks children need those kinds of opportunities provided by the group, rather than because facilities for playschemes happen to be available and no other agency is planning to organise them.

We have noted already that, in the process of clarifying goals, conflicts of interest are likely to emerge within a community group, and these will often be exacerbated as priorities are decided upon. A group may intend to be a multifunctional organisation from the beginning, or it may have formed in order to protest over a single issue 'and in the course of making that protest has established recreational and welfare activities for the sake of raising money and morale and that these activities now seem valuable in themselves' (Baldock, 1974). In both situations, debate about which functions or programmes to concentrate on after an initial phase of activity is likely to bring different interests and viewpoints into overt conflict with each other, and oblige the group to live through a crisis. Baldock also points out that:

where a distinct shift in priorities appears to be required, then this may imply a change of leadership. The leadership thrown up on the first instance may be of people committed purely to one view of what the association should do or with talents that are most appropriate to the initial phase, such as charismatic individuals. It is not uncommon for groups at this stage of development to enter into overt conflict situations in which the early leaders are ejected from their position or alternatively for a group to fail to change its leadership and begin to stagnate. (1974)

An example of the former situation was the decision of community groups which had campaigned against the 1972 Housing Finance Act to continue their existence in a new form when the campaign was over. In the case of the Batley advice centre for the town, this resulted in the falling away from the centre of the most active campaigner against the Act, and a decision by the centre to become a more broadly based advice centre and to seek funds for its organisation. In other words it reassessed its priorities, in the light of a new situation, and changed significantly in its orientation as a result.

While it is easy to explain the need for groups to identify priorities, to make choices as to what they will do, it is much harder to provide guidelines or models of *how* priorities can be identified. Very often discussing the issues in group meetings can be unrewarding. It can lead to increased ill feeling among group members, and the group can fail to arrive at agreed decisions. For a group to experience such failure at a critical stage in its development can be disastrous and every attempt should be made to prevent it.

We are aware that the nature of neighbourhood work implies a high degree of unpredictability; things happen as a result of a wide range of factors – from how local service agencies are perceived by residents, to the intuitions of activists and worker. Nevertheless, there do exist models and techniques developed in other disciplines which can be adapted and used to help community groups reach decisions and make choices about action and programmes. These are worth examining by neighbourhood workers and community groups – even if they subsequently decide to reject them – in order to tighten up on this crucial but weak area of organising. For example, two techniques of which we have had experience are the *nominal group technique* and the *Delphi technique*. We propose to summarise these here but we advise workers to plan to use them to (a) study the original source material and (b) consider how they might adapt the material to their particular situations.

Nominal Groups

The nominal group technique developed from social psychology studies by Delbecq and Van de Ven offers:

a planning sequence which seeks to provide an orderly process of structuring the decision-making of groups, fragmented in terms of vested interests, rhetorical and ideological concepts, and differentiated expertise, needed to be brought together in order for a programme to emerge or change to take place. (1971)

This suggests its possible appropriateness for community groups facing the kinds of choices we are discussing. It is a group process model for situations where there exists uncertainty or possible disagreement about choices, and it can be used for (a) identifying strategic problems and (b) developing appropriate and innovative programmes to solve them. It originated from studies of decision meetings and programme planning in a community action agency during the United States War on Poverty.

The model contains five phases, and for each phase there are specific group techniques and specific roles for different interest groups. The phases are: problem exploration, knowledge exploration, priority development, programme development and programme evaluation. One of the objectives is to facilitate innovation and creativity in planning. Its reliance upon nominal groups (groups in which individuals work in the presence of one another but remain silent) builds upon research studies which indicate the superiority of such groups compared with conventional 'brainstorming' and discussion groups.

Two other important features of the technique are, first, the separation of 'personal' from 'organisational' problems: a large meeting is divided into groups of six to nine people, and each individual is asked to write 'personal feelings' on one side of a card and 'organisational difficulties' on the other side. The person managing the exercise then asks all members of the groups to spend thirty minutes listing aspects of the problem on their cards without speaking to anyone. He then asks one person from each group to record on a common sheet written comments of the members of each group. The groups are then given thirty minutes to review their lists – they can clarify, elaborate or defend any item; or add items. Each member is then asked privately to vote on the five items he considers most crucial on the 'personal' problem list: this represents the end of the first phase of the technique. The remaining four phases require a similar form of structuring.

A second notable feature of the technique is the use of the round-robin procedure which allows each group member to offer an idea; as a result, less secure members will feel more able to follow the risk-taking of more secure members.

The nominal group process provides both quantitative data in the sense of voted-upon priorities and qualitative data in terms of a rich, descriptive discussion which follows the nominal group activity, in which members often provide critical incidents or personal anecdotes.

While the technique relates more obviously to professional groupings (we have made use of it when helping social work teams to decide whether or not to 'go patch'), its methods are also very relevant to community groups, and use has been made of them by neighbourhood workers. It deliberately and systematically structures the business of deciding upon priorities. The point to stress is the need to adapt and modify the technique as developed by Delbecq and Van de Ven (1971) to suit both a community work context and specific situations. We would certainly not advise uncritical transfer of the technique from the social planning context described by the authors to a neighbourhood work setting.

Dephi

A similar hesitation must apply to use of the Delphi technique. It aims to develop scenarios based on expert knowledge of related topics.

The technique is no more than a device which can be used when the agreement of 'experts' on an uncertain issue is desired. Although it originated in forecasting and futurist opinion-gathering it has also been used in industrial decision-making, educational planning and studies in the quality of life. It is claimed to be a 'rapid and relatively efficient way to "cream the tops of the heads" of a group of knowledgeable people'.

Its three main features are anonymity, controlled feed-back and statistical group response. It focuses primarily on identifying items of dissatisfaction among participants:

> In using the method, anonymity is effected through question-naires or other formal communication devices. This reduces the effect on the group that might be produced by dominant individuals. Controlled feedback is used to reduce noise usually encountered in face-to-face conferences. The exercise is conducted as a sequence of rounds in which the results of the previous rounds are fed back to the participants. The statistical group response is a device to assure that the opinion of every member of the group is represented in the final response. (Molnar and Kammerud, 1975)

Although the highly structured nature of the Delphi technique, and its emphasis on the role of the expert, may appear alien to the style and values of community work, it would be short-sighted for workers to dismiss it and other similar techniques out of hand. Most of them have been tested and shown to produce measurable benefits, particularly in situations where a large number of people have to work on complex and ill-defined problems. Local people are knowledgeable about their community, and it is axiomatic that their expertise should be used in the process of reaching decisions about what issues to work on. The Delphi method is simple in concept and there is a great deal of latitude in the specifics of carrying it out.

The 'Neighbourhood Action Packs' developed by Gibson and contained in his book *People Power* (1979) aim to assist groups in ways similar to the two techniques we have referred to. They consist of a range of written and visual materials designed to help groups wanting to 'get at the facts', 'involve the membership' and 'streamline decision-making'. One section is about deciding priorities and taking action, and suggests quick ways to establish general agreement on what needs to be done first, how easy or complicated each issue is likely to be, what kind of action ought to be taken and who should take it. There is material too in *The Community Workers' Skills Manual* (ACW, 1979) which is directly relevant to priorities-setting. The technique entitled 'clarifying what people would like to see happen', like the nominal group technique summarised above, encourages individual members of a group to work on their own for short periods.

Issues For The Worker

At its more exhilarating and turbulent moments the unfolding of a piece of neighbourhood work can appear to be self-evident. The cry from the heart of the worker that his or her job is to 'get out there and organise' is persuasive, and at such moments advice or training guides about the need to clarify role can seem both dampening and restrictive, as well as contrary to the natural instinct of a worker.

Yet, how often has inadequate reflection upon role at different phases in a group's existence contributed to confusion or conflict both for the worker and the group? Too frequently, in our experience. The need for consideraton to be given both to conceptualisation about worker issues and to specific action is, we believe, particularly pressing when, as it were, a group is 'coming of age': it has set itself in a particular direction, it knows what it seeks to achieve. It has gone past the earlier phase of forming itself into a group, and it is not yet faced with problems of maintaining itself or providing services. This 'growth' period of a group should prompt a worker to re-examine his or her own contribution and tasks.

Role

In Chapter 4 we used the term 'role predisposition', because we think a worker's decision about role should be determined partially by the situations in which he and a group find themselves. In that a group has acquired evident strength and sense of purpose, it will often be appropriate for the worker who has given it considerable support to begin to adopt a lower profile, to *appear* to be less intensely involved with the group. He will stop doing so much for the group. He will also seek to establish other ways in which he can help the group in the future. It may be, for example, that a group has decided to develop a welfare rights service and the worker may have limited experience or knowledge in that area. His strength may lie more in being able to offer educational expertise. He should feel able to discuss such a situation openly with the group, and indicate the kind of support he can best offer in the future. He cannot be a jack-of-all-trades, and he is also likely to have other work to do.

Framework for Action

Effectiveness of a worker or a project will be undermined if insufficient work has been put into establishing how the worker will relate to a group once it becomes active. Use of the social work term 'establishing a contract' is not always appropriate in a community work setting, whether it is used in a 'strong' or 'weak' sense, and we prefer to think of a process of open discussion or negotiation as the means by which a future working relationship is agreed upon. Neighbourhood work has, in our view, to remain a fluid and flexible activity; to refer to establishing a contract, even though it may not mean a written contract, is to risk injecting an element of artificiality and rigidity into natural human relationships.

On the whole, people who are active in their community do not want to be pinned down in terms of their precise personal commitments. A worker should never be in the position of appearing to control the rate of activity of a group or the ups and downs of its existence. Whatever method a worker and a group feel most comfortable with, our chief concern is to stress the importance for the worker and the group to decide what kind of support he or she will provide, how frequent it will be, and on what issues or areas of interest it will concentrate. We discuss what these can be in the next chapter.

Naturally, workers will continue to 'care' for the group, and do things for it, outside any formulated agreement, and fulfilling such a role can continue to be very time-consuming. Groups will continue to face internal crises of one kind or another, and a worker will either be asked to help or will feel he needs to offer guidance or support if the group is to survive. It is not easy to divide up a worker's relationship with a group, and in advocating the advantages of setting out a framework of action between worker and group we do not wish to deny the need at times for both parties to go outside it.

Constraints on Workers

If a worker is faced with clear constraints in his job then it is wise for him to explore with the group what these imply. Just as the extent to which workers have discussed with their own agency what they intend to do will be tested as the pressures of work increase, so too understanding by a group of a worker's action in moments of crisis of the group with other organisations will be facilitated if he or she has examined the general question with the group earlier. Our concern here is not to debate the question of to whom a worker owes loyalty and accountability but to suggest that it constitutes an item for discussion between a worker and a group at this stage.

Recording

We draw attention to the need for a neighbourhood worker to have decided upon a manageable and relevant form of recording from the moment that he begins a community project; Baldock has pointed out that many workers write up a neighbourhood analysis, based on their impressions and recordings, after about six months, and recording the progress of a group's formation is vital. However, writers who have discussed recording in community work draw attention to the need for a worker to adopt a well organised recording system once he or she is working with a group on a continuing basis. They also indicate the advisability for workers to limit the amount of recording they do.

Baldock lists four questions a worker should have in mind when doing process-recording of a group, that is observing and noting, for example, the interactions of a group meeting:

Did the group session achieve its purpose?
What was the feeling of the meeting like?
What were the different roles of individuals?
What was the worker's role?

In deciding what kind of recording to do, it can be helpful for the worker to ensure that he does not rely on one method only. The most usual approach is to do narrative-recording, on a day-to-day basis, and to mix this with recording under specific headings. If a worker is part of a team, or if he collaborates closely with workers in neighbouring areas, it is possible to agree what the headings should be and what data should be included under them. This offers an opportunity for comparative studies.

Usually, too, a worker will want to undertake his own recording, to be used essentially to help improve his practice and to provide a basis for evaluation, and a more limited recording for his agency. An example of choosing how to record is taken from a report of a student working on the Southwark Community Project:

> Decision to write report on visit to 'Hole in the Wall' pub. This was a decision involving the use of records. Decided against putting the report in my diary. Because of what it contains felt it would be more relevant as an agency report. Decided that diary should be kept for day-to-day occurrences without too much detail. Did however put incident of man met after leaving 'Hole in the Wall' in diary as this did not occur in circumstances set up by me, i.e. it was just an incident, presumably fairly common in Southwark of being stopped and asked for money. (Thomas, 1976)

Whatever kind of recording workers do they will need to respect the feelings of the group with whom they are working: they should keep detailed recording of the group confidential, and they should only release information about the group for storing in the agency's records with the agreement of the group.

Once again, the need for workers to talk this and other worker-related issues through with the group is underlined. So, too, is the way in which worker skills relate to each part of the neighbour-hood process – they are in use at different times and with varying emphases. Here we have tried to show how recording by a worker can help a group to set priorities.

Standing Back

We conclude by encouraging workers to keep a close watch on the tempo and ideals of a group. They may well have to urge a group to step aside from its involvement in action in order to reflect upon where it is going, to stand back occasionally and consider what members' activity means in relation to the group's goals. At the same time they may need to remind a group of what it can hope to achieve, to share with it their imagination of an improved state of affairs. Neighbourhood workers need to have a visionary and optimistic quality, and it can be useful for them to share this enthusiasm with a group as it struggles to make impact on a local or wider context.

In itemising the above issues which relate to this stage of the neighbourhood work process we have made a somewhat artificial distinction between the launching of an autonomous group and its subsequent continuation. This reflects our concern to 'sharpen up' the identification of specific skill areas for different phases of community organising. In the next chapter we explore the roles and tasks of the worker when maintaining a community group, and many of these will complement the points we have discussed in this chapter.

CHAPTER 8

Keeping the Organisation Going

Providing Resources and
Information
Being Supportive
Co-ordinating Help
Planning
    Policy planning
    Operations planning

Developing Confidence and
Competence
    Technical tasks
    Interactional tasks

Many workers learn the hard way that community groups can be fragile. The seemingly confident group that launched itself with a blaze of publicity may plod on ineffectually, its meetings becoming more and more ritualised. Community action is often a long process, and achievements are rarely immediate. Consequently, a group becomes at risk as interests decline, personal disputes and needs obtrude, and the lack of progress demoralises. Slowness and indifference in the response of a local authority to letters from a newly formed group can sometimes be enough to ensure its withering away.

The maintenance and strengthening of the community group must be an essential interest to the worker and, indeed, to the members and officers of the group. We write 'interest' because there will be some groups who will flourish without anyone 'doing anything' about their development; on the other hand, there are many groups who may fall into dire straits if the worker has not been working hard with members to help the group stay intact and develop. The strength of the group, and the confidence and competence of its members, are thus legitimate matters of concern for the neighbourhood worker, whose contribution to group management has been described by Barr:

A group can, however, only effectively use the knowledge it acquires if it maintains its own internal cohesion and stability.

In deprived areas residents experience many pressures and internal divisions within the community which may be reflected in the way that group members behave towards one another. Indeed, some groups may be so torn by internal divisions that they are never able to represent effectively the interests of their area. Given that this is so, the enabling process within community work is centrally concerned with holding the disparate elements of groups together, and encouraging the group to adopt a collective view of its goals and methods which reflect the needs and views of the area as a whole. This role is often extremely time-consuming and exacting but is an essential prerequisite to effective work by groups. In many respects it is the skill of a community worker in this role that is most important in determining the success of the community work process, yet it is the role which is least visible to outsiders (1977).

Tasks such as helping the group get through a depression or crisis, or assisting individuals to learn new skills and develop in a particular office in the group, may be best approached through understanding the roles the worker takes on, and the force of his or her own personality, energy and enthusiasm in motivating members. It is often the quality of the worker's relationships, and the strength of his own commitment to the group's work, that contribute most to the task of helping to maintain the organisation.

It is possible to provide a number of different ways of conceptualising the group maintenance tasks of the neighbourhood worker. While there is some overlap between them, each can contribute to a particular dimension of the task. For example, the Waychester Project report distinguishes between socio-economic and task functions in area-based work; and describes the former as passing through the stages of establishing/choosing groups and relating to leaders; inspiring; and building genuine self-sufficiency (Taylor *et al.*, 1976).

Group maintenance may also be portrayed in terms of theories about small group behaviour: two researchers refer to 'the ability to work effectively in both small and large groups ... to help people organise themselves into a group and to work towards their goals. It also includes skill at understanding group processes and dynamics.' They quote a community worker as saying:

Just the plain nuts and bolts of getting a group together, helping them to communicate their intentions and their needs ... helping people to present the essentials of their work and their activities, to pitch their communications ... I think there are skills in clarifying with groups what they're for and what you as a community worker are there for. (Thomas and Warburton, 1977)

Thus the 'group work' perspective emphasises the dynamics of the group, as well as the phases or stages of growth through which the group might progress. Brager and Specht (1973), for example, describe group development in terms of four stages and indicate the kinds of tasks for the worker that are present at each stage. McCaughan, too, has written about groups in a paper for community workers, and she discusses different features of group life and organisation (1977b). One of the most useful texts on group work that is available for the neighbourhood worker is that of Ken Heap, published in 1985.

Another slant on the tasks of group maintenance is implicit in those descriptions of the worker's role that stress facilitating, enabling, supporting and encouraging as appropriate behaviours for workers. Murray Ross describe the tasks of the enabling role as focusing discontent; encouraging organisation; nourishing good interpersonal relations; and emphasising common objectives. The worker helps the group to work by contributing calmness and objectivity; a focus on common goals; and an 'analysis and treatment of the causes of tension to the degree that he and the group are able to handle them'.

Ross suggests that the contribution of the worker towards group development is not limited to being helpful in times of crises, disputes and various other impediments to co-operative work. The contribution is essentially ongoing and creative and at its best will help to foresee impending problems and avoid the need for crisis intervention. The nature of this continuing contribution is described by Ross in the following passage:

The professional worker seeks also to increase the amount of satisfaction in interpersonal relations and in co-operative work. He is a warming congenial influence in group and community meetings. This implies a warm, friendly person, sensitive to the deeper feelings of people, and interested in the 'little things' that are important in the lives of individuals and communities. He is concerned with meetings in which people feel comfortable, enjoy themselves and feel free to verbalise. To this end he is alert not only to the physical and psychological conditions which make for such comfort, but seeks to create these conditions and uses his own self to facilitate these. This means he is adept not only in room arrangements, introductions, casual conversations, but that he is sensitive to the process of interaction which goes on in a group and knows when and how to ask that question which will catch and focus the interest of the group, when to interpret what is being attempted, when to praise. People can enjoy working together when they begin to know one another and sense what they can do co-operatively. Part of the worker's role is to assure such satisfaction for the group. (1967)

Ross's chapter on the role of the professional worker is a valuable contribution to our understanding of the tasks of the worker with local groups. Unfortunately, Ross tends to convey a picture of the neighbourhood worker as an angelic figure, moving with ease through the urban 'interpersonal underworld', suffusing light, reason and good-will. It is this flavour in his book that often deters readers from attending to what is probably one of the clearest expositions of those aspects of role that are concerned with the social and emotional needs of a group.

Another view of group maintenance pays attention to the task rather than the socio-emotional elements of group life; the major concern for the worker is with how the group functions as a work and decision-making system. The worker is interested in the effectiveness of the leaders of the group, its levels of participation and recruitment, and the extent to which it is or is seen to be representative of its constituency. The worker is most often seen as a 'resource and information person', feeding into the group concrete data and resources rather than more tangible assistance with, for example, disruptive aspects of the group dynamic.

This kind of conception of the worker's contribution to the work of the group often goes hand-in-hand with a concern to educate politically – for instance, see John Benington's account of the CDP contribution to the Gosford Green Residents' Association (1975). This somewhat austere portrait of the worker as a provider of information, resources and political ideas is in strong contrast to that, for example, provided by Murray Ross.

Education in its broadest sense is at the heart of the work in group maintenance, and provides the final dimension that we wish to discuss in this brief introduction. We have already referred in this book to the distinction between *outcome* and *process* goals. The former refer to the largely material end results of a group's activities, and the latter to the educative aspects of work through which both the group and individual members acquire competence and confidence in a number of skill and knowledge areas. The development of a group, and the learning and change that occurs in individuals, are naturally not confined to those tasks that are to do with group maintenance; nevertheless, it is the tasks of group maintenance that provide by far the greatest challenge and opportunities for learning and it is thus appropriate to refer to the educative aspects of involvement in community action in this chapter.

There are a variety of ways in which process goals are described. For example, some theorists and practitioners are essentially concerned with the development of knowledge and skills in those activities that need to be carried out if the group is to function effectively and achieve its goals. This will be more fully discussed later in the chapter, and they include the development of leadership potential, skills in negotiating and bargaining, and competence in tasks such as running meetings, keeping minutes and accounts, planning, and the execution of group decisions. It is also expected that as individuals learn and extend their skills they will acquire more confidence in themselves, and there will be a development and broadening of the individual's personality, experience and life goals. This may be made manifest not only through the activities of the group but also in the individual's relationships and achievements in settings like his or her family and work. Schler (1970), for instance, has suggested that membership of community groups is intra-psychically beneficial and promotes interpersonal competence, though he gives as much importance to developing the special skills needed to carry out the work of the group. The 'therapeutic' and personal growth qualities of community action and protest are also referred to by Alinsky in *Rules for Radicals* and extensively discussed by Haggstrom (1970).

There are differences between writers and between practitioners in the importance that they give to that development of individuals that occurs *over and above the enhancement of those skills needed for task performance in the group*. The Biddles, for instance, give emphasis to the development of the whole individual; they see community work as a 'group method for expediting personality growth'. This view of community work – which Khinduka (1975) criticises as the psychological approach to social problems used essentially by caseworkers practising in a community setting – is also reflected in those schemes for participation that emphasise the therapeutic aspects of participation rather than the instrumental ones that give value to the social and political benefits of power-sharing.

A different approach to individual change is one that gives most priority to the development of those skills that are needed to push forward the work of the group, and that give the individual the confidence and competence eventually to take part in wider community and city issues. Community workers who take this line accept that changes also occur that benefit the individual in his relations in the family and at work; but these changes are seen as 'spin-offs' that are to be welcomed but are not to be given priority, do not provide the basic rationale for neighbourhood work and should never impede the work of the group in achieving its goals. People do change as a result of being involved in community action, but such changes are ultimately valued because they facilitate, rather than justify, the work of the neighbourhood group.

It would be wrong to end this discussion without referring to those conceptions of process goals that tend to use the language of 'consciousness-raising'. The vocabulary of this view of process is that of enhancing political awareness, and the raising of consciousness, so that people become better able to understand and question those factors that perpetuate poverty and powerlessness. Here again there are differences of emphasis. There are those in community work who would see local people's involvement in neighbourhood groups ultimately justified by gains to be made in political understanding; action at a neighbourhood level might be criticised for being divisive and parochial, but acceptable so long as it deepens participants' awareness of the political and economic predicament of the working class, and prepares them for some eventual systematic confrontation with power-holders. Community workers and projects holding this view would, as O'Brien discusses in the context of the United States New Left, define the process of learning about politics and organising as more important than the achievement of specific goals.

A different emphasis is given by those who stress the value in its own right of neighbourhood action, and the importance to local people of short-term gains and resources. Political learning is then valued in so far as it facilitates the work of the group, and helps individuals become involved in issues and problems outside their community. Such an involvement might just as well be reflected in membership of local political parties and turn-out at government and trade union elections as in the development of a critical class-consciousness. This position may imply a continuum of consciousness along which individuals may progress; the value of such progress is seen to lie primarily in the benefits to the work of the group rather than in the importance of political learning in its own right.

The significant points on this continuum include:

(1) Awareness of the self and one's position and abilities to achieve some change. This includes the emergence of a motivation to seek the change. We have already referred to such changes in the sections on reflection and vision in a previous chapter, and they are discussed by Haggstrom (1970) and Goodenough (1963).
(2) Awareness of the collective aspects of a problem; that is, there are other people going through a similar situation or experience. Schler has described this aspect of raising consciousness as a broadening of the *scope of concern*.
(3) Awareness, not just of the possibilities of collective action, but also of the powerfulness of the efforts of a group as compared to those of individuals. Individuals begin to assess the costs and benefits to themslves and to the community of engaging in a co-operative struggle around some local issue.
(4) Awareness of the political nature of decisions made in places like local government bureaucracies about resources, opportunities, and power-sharing. 'Political' is used here to refer to the process of negotiating and bargaining that occurs over the allocation of scarce resources, and involves the key people or

departments seeking to gain control over resources and power. Discussions between and decisions by elected members are only one aspect of the political process that occurs within local authorities.

(5) Awareness of how the interests and concerns of one's own group relate to those of other groups in the neighbourhood, the local authority or the city. This awareness may reflect a strategic need to form alliances with others in order to achieve change, or the realisation of the need to avoid a situation where groups are competing with each other for the limited resources held by the various government bureaucracies.

Points 4 and 5 on the continuum seem together to define a state of 'community-consciousness' in which people have a political awareness that is bounded by the issues of concern in the local community. They come to see how their lives are affected by these issues, and to understand the powerful grip that local authority bureaucracies have on the lives of working-class families. This community-consciousness may be viewed as akin to the 'factory-consciousness' described by Beynon in his analysis of the shop stewards in the Ford plant at Halewood:

> Politics is basically about power. About who does what to whom. Viewed in this way it is obvious that these men had quite a developed political understanding. The boundary of this politics, however, was the factory floor. It knew about the bosses and the bureaucrats. About exploitation and being screwed. And this knowledge manifested itself in periods of sustained militancy. But it was a politics that was not easily transferable to other areas of class exploitation and power. (1975)

(6) Awareness and interest in broader political and socio-economic issues, for example, in regional, national and international matters. Such awareness may lead to a new or renewed feeling of responsibility that may be reflected in participation in activities like elections and membership of political groups and parties.

(7) Awareness of the world that goes beyond an interest in wanting to know what is going on. The individual develops a

critical appreciation of his position and that of his peers in society, and explores *causal* questions about the arrangements that govern matters like the distribution of income, wealth, opportunities and power.

The members of a neighbourhood group will be at different stages on this continuum, each of which is worthy of respect in its own right, and each of which contributes to the work and potential of the group. The effect of this contribution need not necessarily be always helpful – a group may be deflected in its task both by new members who are at the early stages of consciousness, and by more 'experienced' members who persist in raising 'fundamental' issues before the rest of the group is ready to deal with them. The essential point is that it is certainly not *necessary* (though ideologists may view it as desirable) for any of the members of a community group to develop more 'advanced' states of consciousness in order for that group to achieve its goals. Politically 'unaware' people do participate in groups that achieve much for their constituency and neighbourhood.

We wish now to develop a more detailed account of the tasks that face the neighbourhood worker in helping to maintain and strengthen the community group. We describe below the five major categories of activity of the worker. They are:

(1) providing resources and information;
(2) being supportive;
(3) co-ordinating help;
(4) planning;
(5) developing confidence and competence.

Providing Resources and Information

In order to carry out their work effectively community groups need a variety of resources and a way of gathering and processing information. The worker is an important, but not the only, element in the provision of both resources and information. Ross has described this as the 'expert' role of the worker, providing data and direct advice in such areas as community diagnosis, research skill, information about other communities, advice on methods of organisation and procedure, technical information, and evaluation and interpretation 'of the process of co-operative work which is being carried on'.

As we noted earlier in the chapter, some workers may see the role of providing resources and information as the only one that is legitimate and desirable, and the one that accounts for most of the worker's time and energy. Other accounts of community work, however, set the role of information- and resource-provider together with other roles. Ross, for example, suggests that the role has to be played alongside those of guide and enabler; the YVFF Waychester project describes it as one of several socio-emotional and task functions.

Providing Resources

The word 'resources' has increasingly become a cover-all word and is used in a variety of ways to label a diversity of functions and activities. We use it to refer to the material facilities and aid that a worker can provide for a group. The worker may not be able directly to provide all such resources (nor deem it desirable that she do so) but the worker will be a point of access or of information about them. The kinds of resources we have in mind include the following:

(1) *Basic servicing or administrative resources* that the group needs to do its work. These include secretarial and clerical help, telephone, typewriter, note paper, duplicator, photocopier, files, records and word-processor. In addition to these, a group may also need from time to time resources like transport and a variety of 'plant' that is needed for specific events such as jumble sales, meetings and parties.

(2) *Accommodation* for committee and group meetings, for holding events, and for running particular services, for example, a weekly advice and information surgery. The matter of premises was discussed in Chapter 7.

(3) *Money* to finance the day-to-day costs of the group's work, and also any special projects it wishes to run such as a summer playscheme. The worker may not only advise on where to obtain funds but also be a point of access and facilitation to agency or local authority sources of funds. Many workers also have their own 'seed money' with which to help the starting of groups.

(4) *People.* Most community groups will require volunteers to

take part in specific activities; and specialists (e.g. lawyers) to advise them on certain aspects of their work. Other kinds of specialists might also be needed, such as local craftsmen to carry out some work for the group, and celebrities to attend and open a group function such as a bazaar.

(5) *Special resources* that a group needs to undertake one-off tasks; for example, video equipment, silk-screen printing, tape recorders and so on.

Providing Information

The kinds of information that the neighbourhood worker provides or helps in providing may be seen to consist of the following:

(1) *Basic information.* The range of such information is wide; it includes that considered above about resources as well as data on, for example, the local authority, facts and figures on the community, and on substantive areas of knowledge in fields like housing, planning and welfare rights. It also includes information on matters such as keeping accounts; preparing a press statement; opening a bank account; keeping minutes, and so forth. It is extremely difficult to convey the scope of the information that most workers will be called upon to give, or know where to find.

(2) *General advice.* Here the worker helps in advising on the pros and cons of various issues and courses of action, and in predicting the costs, benefits and general outcomes of matters like new legislation, decisions and events that affect the work of the group. The worker might advise, for example, on the effects of new arrangements for the submission of grant aid applications or on a change a group wants to make in its constitution; or on whether it should register as a charity or not. The worker's advice is sought and given, but he does not expect it to have a special status in the group and it must be considered alongside that of other members.

(3) *Interpretation and analysis.* There is often a role for the worker in helping a group to understand the details and implications of, for example, various proposals and documents such as planning applications, new legislation, data on the community like that in the census or from a special suvey, perhaps done by the group, and 'difficult' letters from officers in the local authority that are replete with jargon, unfamiliar language and style, and vagueness.

Thus workers have to have skills in gathering, interpreting and presenting information in the three distinct but overlapping areas described above. For some kinds of information there are usually guidelines available that the worker might use – for example, on how most effectively to present statistical data to people who may not be numerate. In general, the worker has to consider the presentation of information in terms of how much is given; its timing; its form and style; the medium through which it is conveyed; the characteristics of the people who want it; and the use to which it will be put by them. The reader might consider, for example, how one would take these factors into account in responding to a request from a newly formed tenants' association in a homeless families block 'for a couple of model constitutions'.

The task of providing information and resources appears straightforward, although demanding of a good deal of the worker's time, skills and integrity. It is, however, not without its pitfalls. There are the two related issues of learning and control. It is in the role of information-giver that workers most frequently experience the dilemma of how helpful they should be to a group. If, for example, a group wants a list of local authority committee chairpersons, the worker might suffer considerable anguish in deciding whether he should provide it himself (the quickest solution) or work with members of the group in getting hold of the information (longer, but adds a little to the skill and knowledge of the group).

The other dilemma occurs because of the association of information and access to resources with power and control. Through the selective withholding and giving of information a neighbourhood worker can unfortunately create opportunities to influence the work of a group. She may have the best motives in doing so; she may be right in her assessment that a certain piece of information would only distract the group from its task. But she may be aware that to withhold the information is also to withhold the opportunity for the group to decide on its relevance, and thus to undermine its authority.

Finally, we wish briefly to mention a further problematic aspect of the role of information/resource person. It is that the role offers the opportunity to the worker to establish herself as a go-between, mediating between the group and other organisations and decision-makers in the local authortiy. Even if the worker does not take these opportunities, her involvement in information exchange may lead to her being perceived and responded to as a go-between. The role of go-between is, of course, a recognised one in community work though it is also rejected as being inappropriate by many workers on the grounds that it diminishes the responsibility and authority of the group.

Being Supportive

One of the neighbourhood worker's tasks is to be supportive both of the group and of its individual members. The group particularly needs the support and encouragement of the worker at times when its energies and enthusiasm are low, and it feels it has suffered setbacks, or achieved little, in reaching its goals. The worker can often be supportive in such times by maintaining the interest, optimism and commitment that seem to be waning in group members. He or she attempts to re-galvanise and re-motivate participants. But support of the group should also be on-going, and the worker can provide it by indications of his recognition and respect of its work. These indications or signs may be made manifest in a number of ways, and these have been discussed by Goetschius (1971).

Support for the group is also given when the worker helps its members to assess and evaluate its work, assisting them to see the positive and creative aspects of what they have done. It is given, too, by the worker ably carrying out the work he has offered, or been given, to do on behalf of the group; by attendance and helpfulness at its meetings and neighbourhood events; by 'mucking-in' and taking a share of the routine and boring side of the group's activities; and by being a figure of continuity during those periods when the group is going through changes associated with the loss or the recruitment of members.

There are a number of ways in which the worker gives support to *individuals* of a community group through, for instance, being supportive of individuals learning and experimenting in new roles, such as chairman or treasurer; and of those learning new and challenging tasks. The worker will help individuals to confirm their feelings of competence about new roles and tasks, and about their contributions to the work of the group. Some members of a

240

group might also expect the worker to help them to assess the costs and benefits of their remaining involved in collective action, discussing for example, 'whether the caretaker really can throw me out if I don't give up being secretary'. Such support could as much involve helping individuals leave a group as supporting them to persevere.

In this respect, it is important to note that some individuals may call upon the worker for support and advice about problems in their family or work, or with agencies like the police and the courts. This support may be very tangible indeed, such as asking the worker to stand bail or act as a guarantor to an HP agreement. It is not necessarily only problems with which the worker may be approached; his support may be needed for new endeavours that a person wants to undertake, not just in the work of the group but also in the person's job or in some other aspect of community life.

The style in which workers go about their work may also be seen to constitute a source of support to local people. Friendliness, openness and a willingness to be accessible for a discussion even during the hard-pressed moments of a hectic day can contribute support and encouragement.

It is evident in the relationships of many workers to community groups that the support is a two-way affair. Workers may value the opportunity for discussing work matters with local people, or opportunities that are likely to occur in their personal or work lives. In particular, residents may offer feed-back to the worker on how he relates to them, and about the way in which the worker goes about his job. Residents can offer, too, more general support to the worker as they relate to each other in different roles in settings such as the pub.

Co-ordinating Help

No neighbourhood group is, or ought to be, an island unto itself. Groups who are actively engaged in community action, and who want to achieve their goals, will have developed a host of relationships with other groups, individuals, local government and voluntary agencies and community institutions such as the schools, the churches, trade unions and civic and political bodies.

Many of these relationships develop because they provide access to resources and information that the community group needs in its work. A more detailed examination of these external affairs of a group is provided in the next chapter.

The worker has an important role not just in facilitating knowledge of, or access to, these external resources but in helping to co-ordinate their contribution to the work of the community group. Without some planning and co-ordination of the help provided by 'outside' people and groups, a community group may be as much at risk of being hindered and deflected by external help as assisted by it.

We want to discuss the worker's contribution to co-ordinating the efforts of those who, together with the worker and the group, comprise what Pincus and Minahan call the 'action system' (1973). In neighbourhood work this will typically comprise the group, the worker and other individuals engaged by, or attracted to, the group. These 'outsiders' are often referred to as 'experts' or 'specialists' brought in by the group to assist with often limited and one-off aspects of its work. These experts may just as well be local people as professionals from outside the area; they may just as well be experts in manual tasks as in intellectual ones.

This section is, however, largely confined to a discussion of the worker's role in co-ordinating the help of outside professionals such as the lawyer and the housing aid specialist. The Biddles have described this concern of the worker as helping the group to use expert resources without surrendering to them. Many working-class groups battling with complex issues in fields like transportation, inner city redevelopment and housing provision often need competent legal and technical advice. They will rarely be able to buy this advice, but will need to seek out specialists who are sympathetic to their interests and will provide their time and advice for little or no payment. Community groups operating in the vicinity of a university or polytechnic may attract the interest of students or staff members who have, or who are acquiring, the special expertise required by the group.

The use of these outside specialists is not without its costs. So much depends on their ability to 'demystify' their expertise and to present their advice to the group in a way in which its members can understand and use. Specialists, especially those brought in to advise the group on a one-off basis, can unwittingly confuse and

242

undermine group members by the abstractions and detail of their advice, by the way in which it is presented and by the personal manner and style of the advice givers. Experts can too easily succumb to feelings of wanting 'to take the group by the scruff of its neck' where they believe the group is going about things in the wrong way, or too slowly. They may not appreciate or understand the neighbourhood worker's concern that group members have the opportunity to make their own decisions, and to carry them out themselves. Outside specialists may need to be helped to shift away from seeing the group as a 'client' and to perceive the nature of their contribution as a collaborative one – making a shift from what the Biddles call a 'know-it-all' manner to a 'let's-work-this-out-together' procedure.

The activity of the neighbourhood worker in co-ordinating the help of outside experts may be considered in the following way.

(1) Anticipating the needs of a group for specialist help; being able to locate these experts in the community; and assisting the group to interest them in the work of the group.

(2) Helping group members to make the best use of the specialists by providing information on them and their agencies; clarifying as precisely as possible the issues about which advice is needed; and encouraging group members to adopt a questioning or critical stance towards experts.

(3) Familiarising the specialists with the composition, procedures, goals and history of the group, and with the nature of the neighbourhood in which it operates. This may be partly achieved if the group provides access for the specialists to its files and records; but it is just as important for the specialist to 'tune in' to the neighbourhood and the group in informal social settings.

(4) Advising the specialists about their role in the group and drawing their attention to any negative consequences that their contribution may be having. The worker and the group will want to ensure that specialists do not come to dominate, and that the group does not become overdependent on their advice. The authority of group members may gradually and imperceptibly wither in the face of the specialists' mastery of their subjects and the issues confronting the group; or in the face of the enthusiasm, energies and single-mindedness of outsiders like students. The Biddles have also suggested that the community worker can advise the experts before meeting the group 'to be human. They must be

asked to avoid demanding the honour they may think is due to them and the professional manner that invites the honor.'

(5) 'Translating' the advice of the specialists for group members. No matter how well advice has been presented, the worker may need to continue to work with members after the group meetings in order better to understand and clarify the contribution of the specialists, and to assess the implications of that advice for the work of the group and the well-being of its constituency.

(6) Keeping the specialists 'on ice' so that they are ready to respond to the group when it approaches them. This involves the worker in keeping them informed of the work of the group, and securing their continued interest in its affairs. This can be done by the group inviting them to its social occasions and to activities like fund-raising events and annual general meetings. There is a particular role of the worker in securing the continued support of outside helpers when the worker himself has left the group. This is discussed in Chapter 10.

The task of the neighbourhood worker in co-ordinating outside help does not necessarily imply a role of 'go-between' or intermediary. On the contrary, the task of the worker is not to stand as a filter or channel between the group and outside helpers but rather to promote direct and personal contact between them. His responsibility is to make this direct contact as fruitful as possible, and thus to ensure that the use of specialists has a positive impact on the work of the group. The worker's interest in facilitating the interation between group and helpers is to see that group members enhance their own confidence and abilities in finding and using such help. The worker aims for a point in group development where his role in facilitating this interaction becomes less significant.

Planning

It may at first appear incongruous to separate out planning as an activity. It has been an essential aspect of many of the worker's and group's activities that have been discussed in this book. In Chapters 2 and 4, for example, we considered the planning of the community worker's entry and subsequent interventions in a neighbourhood. In Chapter 2 we stressed the importance of planning in carrying out a collection of data about a community. We have also drawn attention to the value of planning for events like meetings and deputations.

We have identified it here as a separate activity largely because effective planning – a concern to anticipate and prepare for future events, and to initiate them – is essential to the maintenance of a soundly functioning and successful organisation. This is particularly the case for neighbourhood groups where a number of factors may conspire to make them over-involved in their present activities and less concerned with what the future holds for them and their constituency. For instance, most residents participate in neighbourhood groups in their spare time; they may have the energies to concern themselves only with the immediate concerns of a group, and insufficient to enable them to plan ahead. Immediate issues may be so pressing and complex and a group's resources so inadequate, that group members are forced to attend to things as and when they happen. In this way, there is often a tendency for neighbourhood groups to do things incrementally, and to be reactive to events in their community, and to the requirements of their own operations.

There appears to be a role for the worker in promoting a concern in the neighbourhood group with two kinds of planning. These are policy planning and operations planning.

Policy Planning

Here the planning is to do with the salient issues and problems facing a group's constituency or the community of which it is a part. This kind of planning will concern some neighbourhood groups more than others; for example, a group set up to oppose the speculative redevelopment of an area, or one set up to deal with employment opportunities, will find it essential to forecast and predict major policy decisions and shifts, and to identify trends in the demography and work patterns of the working and resident population of the community. Such a group may wish to initiate discussion of future issues and events that may not yet have been considered by policy-makers or the general public.

Operations Planning

All neighbourhood groups must attend to this kind of planning if they are to survive and be successful. Operations planning is to do with the group's own administrative and political procedures; it may be said to consist of the following six concerns, the first four of which have been suggested by Schler (1970).

(1) The rational setting of goals and priorities.
(2) Identifying, acquiring and planning the use of resources within and outside of the group so as best to achieve the goals of the group.
(3) A rational process of dividing up labour and allocating work and responsibilities.
(4) The administration and co-ordination of the various subgroups and activities that comprise the neighbourhood group.
(5) Devising and keeping to procedures to ensure that tasks are completed and deadlines met. This involves planning the preparation and submission of, for example, reports to sponsors, applications for funding, petitions to policy-makers and information to constituents. It also involves the kind of detailed planning that is necessary to mount a successful community event such as a summer playscheme.
(6) Preparing the group's tactics and strategies in its negotiations with decision-makers. This comprises discussing which of available tactics are feasible and desirable for the task in hand, evaluating their costs and benefits to the group and trying to assess the likely consequences of particular courses of action.

A word of caution is necessary here. It is not suggested that workers impose planning tasks or frameworks on to groups; rather, they should first listen and observe in order to see any less obvious ways in which a group may be engaged in planning its affairs.

Developing Confidence and Competence

One of the neighbourhood worker's fundamental concerns from the very outset of contacts with local people is to help them acquire confidence and competence in themselves and their abilities to carry out tasks on behalf of the group. It may therefore appear strange that we have highlighted this aspect of the work within the central part of our account of the process of neighbourhood work. We have done so partly because the maintenance of the group is dependent upon the efficient execution of a large number of tasks; and partly because the neighbourhood worker will find that a large proportion of his or her time, energies and skill is needed to help people develop their abilities in the kinds of tasks outlined below.

The neighbourhood worker has the job of helping local people acquire confidence and competence in two broad categories of tasks – the technical and the interactional. We shall consider each separately, though in practice they are intimately connected and often difficult to distinguish.

Technical Tasks

These tasks are often referred to as civic or committee skills. They comprise a wide range of jobs involved in the administration of the affairs of the community group, though not all groups need skills in all technical tasks. Lower-order technical tasks that have to be carried out in most groups include writing letters, keeping accounts, preparing agendas, taking minutes, using the telephone and other items like duplicators, photocopiers, video equipment, and so on, and printing and distributing newsletters. Higher-order tasks include matters such as doing a self-survey, running a petition, leading a deputation, appearing on television and local radio, preparing a press release, organising a rent strike, taking a landlord to court under public health legislation, and objecting to planning proposals at a public inquiry.

We must stress that these are only examples; the nature of the technical tasks will vary with the concerns and issues facing particular groups. But whatever the nature of these tasks, the neighbourhood worker will be heavily engaged in helping people to develop sufficient skills and knowledge to accomplish them.

We are hesitant to use the terms lower- and higher-order technical tasks because we do not wish to imply that the higher-order tasks are necessarily more difficult. Often the contrary is the case: neighbourhood workers will often find themselves spending hours of their time encouraging people in tasks like writing letters or managing finances. It will depend on the experience of individual members of each group whether or not the lower-order tasks are easily accomplished. The amount of time spent by the worker in helping with tasks like writing minutes and funding applications will vary with the experience and background of the individuals concerned. The worker who finds himself spending a whole morning (and perhaps longer) in helping a secretary do the letters that have emanated from the previous evening's committee meeting will often feel very tempted to do the work himself in order to have done with it quickly. The worker can at least expect that if he is doing his job properly then the amount of time he will have to put in on such work will begin to diminish as group members become more skilled and confident.

Although the general rule is that the worker's job is to encourage group members to do the work, there will clearly be some exceptional occasions when the worker finds that he has to do some of the technical tasks himself. Such occasions occur, for example, if the relevant group officer is ill or not functioning in the group because of, say, domestic or work problems. Emergencies often occur (for example, when a group has a week's notice to submit a funding application) and the need for the worker actively to assist in the production of the application will over-ride his own considerations for the learning of group members.

Interactional Tasks

Interactional tasks are of two kinds: first, political skills and competence; and, secondly, caring and supportive capacities within the neighbourhood group.

Group members need to become adept in political transactions within the group, and between the group and the constituency that it represents. The group also has to develop skills in managing its relationships with organisations in its environment – the town hall, service agencies, potential resource people and groups, the press and television, other neighbourhood groups, councillors, MPs, trade unions and public and private industries. Relationships with all these systems require broad political skills in representing, and negotiating for, the interests of the group. It also includes competence in executing and evaluating chosen strategies and tactics.

People who take leadership roles in neighbourhood groups also need to be caretakers of the emotional life of the group, and to be aware of the effects from events in people's personal lives on the group's work. Caring for the group also involves 'training' members for leadership roles, sharing the burden of the work and attending to the recruitment of new members. The neighbourhood worker and leaders need to understand, and mobilise in the group's interest, the original and changing motivations for membership of the group, and to be sensitive to the effect of behaviour in the group like scapegoating. A fuller discussion of the work of the community worker in caring about the group is provided in Thomas's account of the Southwark Community Project (1976). It is clear both that the 'caring' aspects of these interactional tasks encompass many of the points discussed earlier in this chapter in the section called 'Being Supportive', and that there is often a connection between group accomplishment and group members' development. Successful action can often pull people out of their personal antagonisms.

One difficulty in looking at interactional skills from the point of view of individual members is that it may distract our attention away from the group as a system. Groups take on a life and a force of their own that is something more than that given to it by the sum contribution of its individual members. A handbook produced by the Community Projects Foundation warns:

> It is easy to blame whatever is wrong on individuals, but when the same situations crop up in different kinds of groups in different parts of the country, it cannot be individual personalities which cause the problems. Problems in groups are usually caused by bad systems, not by bad people. (1977)

The handbook discusses the interactional (and some technical) aspects of group maintenance in terms of different types of groups, the different stages of group life, aspects of leadership and membership, the purposes of meetings and the different functions and roles that have to be carried out in a group. The handbook suggests 'it is vital to keep an eye on what is happening inside [the group]' because 'if something is wrong with the way a group works, it has much less chance of achieving its aims.'

The theories or models of group change that a worker will use to understand what is going on in a group, and the phases through which it is proceeding, will be determined by a number of factors, not least of which will be their proven usefulness to the worker in helping her in her work. No one way of conceptualising group development is necessarily better or more correct than another. It may be that workers will need to draw upon a variety of explanations about group behaviour according to how they best explain the phenomena present in a group at a particular time.

Neighbourhood workers may use general models and theories about groups that have been the product of thought and investigation in the field of social psychology or group dynamics. McCaughan has provided an introduction to some of these (1977a). There are other views of the development of groups that are the results of research into neighbourhood groups, which have been analysed and written up in order better to understand and enhance community work practice. Two examples are the work of Burghardt (1977) and Zurcher (1972).

Groups change and develop, and it is part of the neighbourhood worker's role to help group members understand that these changes are taking place, and to appreciate their effect on the way individuals are relating to one another and contributing to the work of the group. Many workers are understandably suspicious (see, for example, the 1975 ACW booklet on knowledge and skills) about including a concern wtih group development and dynamics as part of their work. We must stress, therefore, that the role of the worker is 'to keep an eye on what is happening' and to assist group members to understand and respond to the nature of group change and processes. It is not suggested that the worker herself intervenes to bring about substantial changes in the group's life, even if it were possible for her, as a single individual, to do so.

The job of helping people develop skills in technical and interactional tasks demands of the worker time and patience. The availability of time to allow her to work with group members on these tasks is in turn a product of her own ability to manage her workload and not to be so over-burdened that she is unable to find the space in her week to sit down with a group member to help him with the tasks he has been given to carry out. Developing the technical and interactional skills of a group also demands flexibility of the worker in the kinds of role she is prepared to take on.

There will be occasions in the life of a group when its maintenance will hinge on whether the worker is prepared to accept a role (e.g. the post of treasurer) that she would not normally want to have. Another kind of flexibility is that of being able to take on 'missing roles' in the group. The worker may become aware that the work of the group is being hindered because there is no one in the group helping the less confident members to participate; or no one who is clarifying and summarising the points of a discussion as it proceeds. The kind of roles that the worker may temporarily fill, and model for group members, were discussed in Chapter 4 in relation to non-directive role behaviour.

What a worker has to do to keep the organisation going is partly dependent on what happens to the group in its relationship with other organisations. We started this chapter by suggesting that the way in which 'they', the authorities, respond, can critically affect the stability and confidence of a group. In the next chapter we want to look more closely at what is involved for a worker in helping a group in its relationships with organisations such as local authority departments.

CHAPTER 9

Dealing with Friends and Enemies

A delegation from an active tenants' association on a large estate of some 2,500 dwellings meets with members/staff of a local trust.

The tenants are accompanied by a neighbourhood worker who is employed by the borough's social services department and who is responsible for a wider area than the tenants' estate. He is there to support their application to the trust for a grant which will enable them to employ a neighbourhood worker for their estate.

The purpose of today's meeting is for the trust to obtain a clearer idea of the proposed job, before it reaches a decision on the application. It wants to know, specifically, what the neighbourhood worker would do; that is, the trust wants to acquire a better understanding of the roles, tasks and skills involved in doing neighbourhood work. It is also anxious to know why the neighbourhood worker from the Social Services Department cannot continue to serve the estate in addition to the larger area.

The above is a briefing for a role play exercise we have used during training workshops for neighbourhood workers. In addition to testing the ability of workers to articulate what it is they do in neighbourhood work, the role play also forces workers to examine the question of how a community group relates to other groups and organisations in the community. The material focuses on the issue of the planning, tactics and techniques that a group can practise and adopt in order to achieve its objectives; in this example it has to know what the meeting is about, find out who is on the trust committee, send them papers in advance, decide who in the delegation is to speak on particular issues and how best to present the argument. It has also to know what role the neighbourhood worker will play in the meeting.

Giving attention to these kinds of detailed practice questions flows from examination of the theme of 'external affairs' of a group, of how it relates to both friendly and hostile elements of society with which it comes into contact. We shall explore four components of this:

(1) identifying and negotiating with decision-makers;
(2) a group's relationship to other groups and organisations in the community;
(3) a group's own constituency and the public;
(4) the social policy perspective – city, regional and national issues.

A group that has become skilled in its relationship to other systems will often be in a position of having to manage significant financial and human resources. In the final section of this chapter we discuss how the administration and provision of resources or services appear to demand particular skills.

Identifying and Negotiating with Decision-Makers

Action by community groups and neighbourhood workers which relates to influencing decision processes must necessarily draw upon substantial political skills, those which Bryant and Holmes describe as:

Ability to view local initiatives within a broader socio-economic framework of reference, a knowledge of the sociology of political decision-making and a grasp of different varieties of political ideologies and their work within a political framework. (1977)

While knowledge of political and administrative studies is an essential part of neighbourhood workers' training, they need to relate closely to the kinds of issues which are likely to confront neighbourhood groups. An intellectual understanding of political processes has to be combined with practical political skills. We shall see how the ability to 'read a political situation', to think and act politically, are essential prerequisites for a community group and a neighbourhood worker. Without them, neither group nor worker is likely to be effective over a period of time. Nor will their survival chances be high. It is possible to distinguish three contexts of community organising where the political skills of identifying and negotiating with decision-makers are of paramount importance.

Building a Profile of the Target

Whether a group is to have a low-key exchange of opinions with a decision-making body or a tough dialogue over a particular issue, it needs to put time and energy into finding out about that particular organisation: what resources does it have, what is its mandate, what new ideas is it interested in, who does it represent, how is it controlled, what is its constituency? These are broad strategic questions which can be applied to most organisations and which a neighbourhood worker can encourage a group to consider. Clearly, he can share with a group the information he collects when constructing organisational profiles, which we discussed in Chapter 3.

However, the most pointed questions are usually about where power, authority and influence within an organisation lie. Locating these will help a group to present a case, to win allies or to achieve change. Thomas (1978b) refers to the literature on power within organisations and on the potentialities and techniques for low-level employees to wield power and influence within their organisations. Both of these are directly relevant to a community group when it assembles a profile of an organisation. Patti and Resnick identify two important factors for a worker to consider when deciding what change he hopes to achieve within an organisation. He must first:

> examine the agency's decision-making process to determine who exercises both formal authority and informal influence on the outcome of his proposal. In other words, how are decisions made in the organisation on the specific issue in question, and who is in a position to influence this process? . . .
>
> Second, the change agent must consider whether those who exercise formal authority or informal influence in the decision-making process are likely to agree or disagree with his proposal. This kind of analysis is important because it enables the change agent to anticipate how much resistance or support his proposal is likely to encounter. (1975)

A community group which 'sizes up' an organisation, such as a local authority department or a local trust, in this way, is likely to be poised in a far stronger strategic and tactical position than the group which neglects to do so. The neighbourhood worker can play a crucial role here, especially by raising appropriate questions with the leadership of a group.

The other aspect of building a profile of an organisation which a group wishes to influence relates to *how* this can be done. Booklets such as the *Investigator's Handbook*, produced by *Community Action* (1975c) and familiar to many workers, can be valuable guides. Although the handbook's prime concern is to help people needing information about companies, organisations and individuals for campaigns, it is useful for other forms of community organising too. The checklists and suggestions contained within it can be translated by groups and workers to fit particular local situations and, as the handbook takes care to emphasise, these can only be a starting-point from which to build up further investigation and collect different kinds of information appropriate to the needs and strategy of a community group at a particular time.

The above approach must include an attempt to anticipate what effects a group's action will have: 'Whether educating, bargaining, or disrupting, community workers and groups must assess what response or retaliation is possible from the target as they plan their course of action' (Brager and Specht, 1973). Such an assessment can best be made through a concerted and planned effort to find out about and understand the target. Material in a book like Houlton's *The Activist's Handbook*, written for trade unionists, can be transferred to a community group setting in a similar way to the *Investigator's Handbook*. The author's warning to trade unionists is apposite to group members too:

> Understanding how hierarchies operate in organisations should not be the same as saying they are 'right', 'normal', or justified in every situation. The activist should be aware that knowing the rules and using the rules are the first steps in a conditioning process. This knowledge and skill becomes a source of power in itself. So be careful! (1975)

Negotiating by Community Groups

Community groups inevitably use up considerable time and energy in negotiating with decision-making organisations. Cheetham and Hill have pointed out that even conflict strategies

> do not usually imply face to face confrontations of the 'march on the Town Hall', 'sit-in', 'bloody nose' variety. More frequently they involve a process of bargaining and negotiation in an attempt to reach compromise solutions in situations where each party has some real power it can exert over the other. (1973)

Negotiating can usefully be seen as a process in itself, rather than approximating to a once-and-for-all event. For example, an invitation by a group to members of a trust to visit it could be made months before an application for funds was submitted; yet the visit could influence the outcome of the application.

Two essential pre-negotiating tasks for a group are detailed preparation of a negotiating stance, and practice or rehearsal of the case to be put. If a delegation is due to go into a negotiating meeting the roles of its members have to be agreed upon in advance: who will outline the background to the issue, who will supply factual information, who will articulate the group's case, who will respond to offers made across the table? Having decided upon the orchestration of their negotiation, members of the delegation should be encouraged to rehearse it: entering the room, introducing themselves, rearranging the seating to their advantage, working out a signal to request an adjournment during the meeting.

If the idea of anticipating and practising in this way appears excessive it should be remembered that negotiating is not only one of the most significant actions for a group but also often one where it can be most vulnerable. Studies by Dearlove (1973), Newton (1976) and others of local political processes demonstrate the ease with which powerful local authorities can outwit, co-opt or outlast a community group in a protracted negotiating process, and the experiences of many groups tell a similar story. One of the CPF's handbooks (1977) suggests five ways in which local councils and other authorities hold power over community groups: control of resources, control of the timetables, expert knowledge, definition of the problem and access to information. Preparation and practice can offset the power imbalance to some extent, and give leaders of a group or a delegation critical confidence and competence.

Brager and Specht select three priority skills in negotiating by community groups.

Formulating demands	'The outcome of bargaining is determined by the way in which demands are formulated rather than by the merits of the case or by the pressures applied during bargaining.'
Regulating threat	'Threats may be communicated with varying degrees of firmness.'
Reasonableness vs obstinacy	'Reasonableness suggests that a settlement is possible; obstinancy implies that real concessions must be made. This is why negotiating teams sometimes embody both approaches in different team members.' (1973)

The experience and knowledge of labour relations negotiation should not be applied uncritically to the community group context. The latter, after all, normally lacks both the equivalent power and significance of trade union delegations, and it is essential for the form and timing of negotiating by groups to relate to local circumstances. The usefulness of drawing upon negotiating skills in other spheres lies primarily in the techniques and tested experiences which can be borrowed. There are increasing numbers of accounts in community work literature of how groups have negotiated with decision-making or resource-holding bodies. There remains, however, less material which examines the thinking behind negotiating stances of community groups, that is to say, strategy building.

Deciding Strategy

In our experience community groups in the United Kingdom, often under the influence of neighbourhood workers, tend to operate with a relatively simple strategic framework. This may reflect traditional British pragmatism, as well as a tendency for community projects to be composed of a range of interests and political views; the latter is captured in the account by Rustin of the influential 1967 Notting Hill Summer Project:

> Little fundamental discussion took place on this Committee about the general aims and strategy on the Project. There was obviously a diversity of orientations among the members – these were not incompatible in the context of a summer project, but should have been talked through. (1967–8)

Yet the process of talking through differences should not be allowed to stifle the organisation of a project. Groups may have tended to acquire a sharper political focus since the Notting Hill Project and thus approximate closer to their United States counterparts, but their framework is often still expressed in terms of choosing consensus or conflict strategies. They tend not to have as a reference point more complex typologies, such as the one advanced by Brager and Specht (1973).

It should be noted that the nine overlapping strategies distinguished by the Community Development Projects (1974) related to the ideas of CDP staff and the development of each project's strategy, not to the action of the groups with which the projects worked. It would appear that British community work is still experiencing a lag between the articulation of coherent strategies by some workers, based on certain theoretical assumptions, and the sharing and application of them within community groups.

Groups do, of course, carry out effective strategic action in relation to target organisations, but we suggest that they tend to do so implicitly, rather than making explicit use of the language of strategy building whether this be influenced by social psychology or political science. The following questions are central to that process.

What Will the Outcome Be?   Groups need to be clear about the desired end-result of a strategy. In the case of seeking funds, for example, will public or private funding be most appropriate? There is little point in a group engaging in an exhausting struggle for local authority funding if it is clear that the conditions under which a grant is made will be unacceptable and that they cannot be changed.

Equally, a group needs to consider the implications of allowing its strategy to depend too much on one or two external individuals, in case the same persons retain their grip on the group's future once they have helped it achieve a particular goal. An example might be the role of a local authority chief executive officer. In the US Model Cities Program, it was found that the degree of active commitment by a city's chief executive was a crucial determinant of the planning process, which included the involvement of local residents. Do local authority chief executives in this country fulfil a similar function, particularly in facilitating a group's proposal through the decision-making process? A group is wise to look ahead at the possible outcomes of making major use of a strong ally, and weigh up the advantages and disadvantages.

Which Tactics?   A group needs to select the direction of its strategy and then proceed to weave together tactics which support it. Most groups employ both 'inside' and 'outside' tactics, obtaining results by both having allies inside large bureaucratic organisations, and making their presence felt by clever use of resources external to the target organisation – effective publicity being especially important. In their article Cheetham and Hill write of the scope for local groups to achieve change within local government. They note the desire of local elites to achieve some sort of consensus in the community for which they have responsibilities, and how:

Securing influence will be a matter of finding powerful allies, and 'fighting' on an issue will be a complex matter of adopting several strategies at once. In such a situation there may be a separate place for the committed 'insider', the publicity-conscious organisation leader and the mass protest operating all at the same time. (1973)

Who Should Be Lobbied?   Related to the question of political tactics is that of the types of 'resource transaction' implied by an issue or problem: groups, for example, can wish to acquire a certain resource – a community centre, open space, a mini-van – or it can seek to improve the quality of existing resources or services – caretaking facilities, a playground, surgery opening hours. We develop this typology of resource transactions at the end of the chapter. Here we alert the reader to the point that the nature of a neighbourhood worker's support of a group needs to be influenced by the type of transaction being planned by it, becuase certain transactions are likely to require particular personal qualities, attributes and skills.

Opinions voiced by community groups will not be heard by target organisations unless they are presented to influential people in these organisations convincingly and forcefully. The former requires there to be good arguments linked together and supported with valid evidence; the latter requires groups to lobby. Deciding who to talk to, and how best to arrange to do so, can pay dividends in terms of the ability of community groups to achieve their goals.

It is important that lobbying is not perceived as a last-minute effort nor as a sufficient tactic by itself, for then the person or persons being lobbied will feel themselves to be under unacceptable pressures and will also tend to regard those who are doing the lobbying as motivated chiefly by self-interest. If a group has relied for support on one political party in the town hall and made no effort to communicate with other parties, it cannot expect to be listened to by the latter if the group suddenly sees how they could be useful to it.

Lobbying consists of building trust and interest between a group and those with political influence, and this can be demanding on a group's time, patience and resources. Often it involves 'being around' when important meetings take place, and informal talk in canteens and bars. The times when it is possible for a group to do intensive lobbying on a particular issue are comparatively rare, and the effectiveness of such lobbying depends on strong connections having been built up beforehand. Lobbying is an established feature of Britain's political system and there is no reason why community groups should not gain benefits from it. In attempting to do so, however, they should not underestimate the skills required.

What Leverage Do We Have? A stage beyond lobbying is when a group knows that it can bring to bear real threat on a target organisation, and when it is in the interest of that organisation to give in to threat. This is known as leverage. It implies that considerable work has gone into compiling a profile of an organisation, to the extent that its vulnerable areas have been discovered. The effective use of leverage depends upon accurate forecasting of an organisation's actions, so that a group can bring about the desired response.

Probably the most frequent form of leverage deployed in community work, associated with the tactics of Alinsky, is the use of embarrassment which either exposes an agency to public ridicule or undermines the 'professionalism' of agency staff. Examples would be: peaceful demonstration on immaculate lawns surrounding municipal buildings by children demanding play areas; publicising the wealthy residence of a private landlord who refuses to undertake repairs and maintenance of his homes; and exposure of policy contradictions of an organisation through the release of confidential information.

As the last example suggests, making use of leverage tactics can place a group on a moral knife-edge, and any group needs to think carefully about both the ethics and the consequences of employing them; the costs of using leverage can outweigh the benefits if a group is seen to be using manipulative means in public life, since it is these that community work values purport to oppose. And making use of leverage risks leaving a group more vulnerable than before. Leverage can be an ultimate test of how able a group is at gamesmanship when implementing its strategy.

Is the Timing Right? The most important strategic consideration of all for community groups concerns the timing of any action; in some cases this can be even more vital than which issue a group chooses, for skilful timing may have the potential for opening the way for several issues. In terms of having greatest impact on decision-making, a group must aim to become involved in the process as early as possible. Planning and housing issues in particular have to be confronted before authorities take crucial decisions which then allow for only minor modification. The difficulty with early involvement is that it puts a severe strain on the ability of groups to sustain an even level of commitment over a long time. We have noted already how groups tend to become increasingly vulnerable, in a negotiating process, to the pressures of better-resourced and more expert agencies.

The question of timing highlights the role of the neighbourhood worker as a significant source of support for groups as they search for effective strategies with which to influence decision-makers. Taking the position of always acting as a resource to a group demands considerable self-discipline by the worker, well explored by Von Hoffman:

> The best organisers have single-track minds. They care only for building the organisation. When they alienate a potential member they do so out of organisational need, not out of the egotism of irrelevant personal values. The best organisers stifle their tastes, their opinions, and their private obsessions. (1972)

Of the three kinds of representation we referred to in Chapter 4 – observer/recorder, delegate and plenipotentiary – it is the first which a worker usually occupies when a group engages with a decision-making body. For example, it is members of the group who should speak on behalf of a delegation during a meeting. The worker's role should be much more one of helping a group prepare for the meeting. He or she must be adept at calculation, and at encouraging leaders of a group to assess, with tactical acumen, the pros and cons of different approaches before what are often very testing encounters for group members. They should also list the possible alternative stances the group might adopt, such as the following:

(1) *Empathising with the target.* This approach, much favoured by Alinsky, requires group members to comprehend the others' problems, without losing their capacity to present a strong case and to apply pressure. This can suggest where pressure might most

effectively be applied. Political judgement can be increased, too, when a worker can distinguish the professional role or job which a person has to perform from his social role.

(2) *An appearance of reasonableness.* It may be sensible for a group to project a reasonable and responsible image, particularly when it suspects that the target may use alleged unreasonableness or irresponsibility by the group to discredit it. Groups need to guard against helping authorities to ignore their case by attacking the way in which the group presents itself. Paying attention to the question of how to approach an organisation is one way of preventing that outcome.

(3) *Multi-focused strategies.* We indicated above the advantages of developing multi-pronged strategies as opposed to relying on one or two tactics. Yet there may be resistance in a group to that argument, based either on ideological reluctance to 'play the game' of mobilising forces in its favour both within and outside the target organisation, or on a refusal to believe that more than one action arena is necessary at any one time: 'We are going down to talk with the committee' – implying that that by itself will resolve the matter – can be the collective opinion of a group, and a suggestion by the worker that other action needs to be happening at the same time can receive short shrift. In this case, a worker can point to situations where groups have made effective use of multi-focused strategies from which other groups can learn.

Our survey of the skills required by community groups when they are engaged in identifying and negotiating with decision-makers, and the complementary role of neighbourhood workers, has had to be selective. It is a rich area which draws not only on the varied experiences of workers but also on the practice and study of labour relations and politics. Groups and workers will never be provided with blueprints for action in neighbourhood work, but least of all in this topic. They need to develop action appropriate to their goals and to the opportunities of the situation within which they are organising. This last point underlines again the essentially political nature of the skills we have discussed.

Relating to Other Groups and Organisations in the Community

Consideration by neighbourhood workers of the value of helping to form federations of community groups and umbrella organisations has increased in recent years. There is more awareness of the advantages of organising in this way and of the likely implications for community groups. The idea itself, of course, is not new within community organising: councils of social services were formed on the basis of providing a focal point for voluntary organisations in a town or borough, and a number of large community associations have operated on the same principle, usually in a smaller geographical area, for some time. Some of the opportunities and constraints of federations are further discussed by us in an article in the *Community Development Journal* (1981).

Although neighbourhood groups can draw upon well-tried experience when they consider how to relate to other groups and organisations in the community, there is relatively little in community work literature about this form of organising. Both this absence, and perhaps the experiences of federations themselves, suggest that it is so far an underdeveloped area when compared with more usual forms of neighbourhood organising. Ohlin has noted the problems experienced when bringing together a broad range of existing groups in an area as a means of organising indigenous movements:

> Such associations often represent little more than objectifications of the existing power structure in the area. It then becomes exceedingly difficult to secure representation for new indigenous interests in such associations. (1969)

In this country there is tacit recognition of the difficulties and challenges, at the same time that it is seen to be an essential line of development for community work. In *The Teaching of Community Work* the 'third type of group situation' which a community worker will meet is described as:

> that composed of representatives of other organisations. Each member will come owing prior allegiance to his own agency and may have varying degrees of ambivalence to the purposes of the

264

group. Being able to work effectively with such a group is of vital importance at all levels of community work. (CCETSW, 1974)

Such ambivalence has been experienced by many workers who have tried to form borough-wide groupings. An invitation will be given by workers to groups to send representatives to a meeting, yet, as in this example:

Quite a lot turned up, but nothing came out of it. They followed up the meeting with a questionnaire, sent round to get more details of issues important to tenants. No replies came back.

Afterwards, the worker considered that it had been too complicated an exercise, transport problems made regular communications difficult between groups in the borough, they may have been too keen to talk about problems rather than highlight what strengths and experiences people could share with each other, and there was a lack of structure of communication.

Clearly, there are crucial factors to take into account when the idea of a federation is being considered. It is important to estimate the resources of the likely constituent groups, especially the availability of committed and skilful people to work at that level. Workers must judge too how much existing groups will *in fact* have in common, as compared with working together through discussion and sharing of ideas. It will be the priority issues facing a community which will be the major determinants of the form and content of organising.

We consider below how groups tend to come together across an area, and suggest that one way of understanding various experiences is to distinguish between those organisations which originate chiefly from the *practical needs* of community groups and those which form more through realisation of their *common values*. However, we shall see that the results of both these starting-points tend to be similar.

It is important to emphasise that, in concentrating in this section upon federations and umbrella organisations, we do not wish to imply that this is the only way for community groups to relate to each other. It is possible, for example, for groups to keep in touch through exchanges of newsletters, and a worker needs to consider carefully the benefits of this and other options before advising groups to bind themelves together organisationally. Taking such a step is usually a major undertaking for any group, which is why we propose to examine it in more detail.

Practical Origins of Organising Between Groups

Most community groups look to either a defined geographical area or within a local authority boundary when they consider working together. Examples in London have been the coalition of groups in north Southwark to contest the proposals for redeveloping the Coin Street area, and solidarity of a range of groups in the struggle to keep open the Elizabeth Garrett Anderson hospital for women at Euston. Town-wide and city-wide organisations have been formed around different issues and problems.

Play is an activity which often leads to the formation of umbrella organisations. Playgroups, holiday playscheme committees and adventure playground projects can all frequently appreciate the benefits of joining with groups which have similar interests. It enables them to co-ordinate their activities, which can be particularly important when several groups share one resource such as a minibus, and it can provide an essential framework for securing future funding. Many tenants' and residents' associations have also realised the practical gains they can obtain by establishing an umbrella grouping, either on a borough-wide basis or covering a smaller area, such as three neighbouring estates.

Indeed, it is possible to find examples of most kinds of community work activity which have spawned co-ordinating mechanisms of one sort or another. Astin (1979) describes how the Barton Information and Advice Centre linked up with other centres in the Oxford Area, in order to support each other, develop their effectiveness (particularly through training) and to pursue common objectives. The authors of *Resources for Social Change* (Glen, Pearce and Booth, 1977) include a case study of how the Cumbria CDP helped to set up a day centre for the elderly and they record how the example demonstrated the value simply of bringing different groups together which have a common interest.

Sometimes it will be community groups, supported by a worker, which will take the initiative to organise together. At other times, as in the Cumbria example, it will be a project or worker who proposes such a strategy. Brager and Specht's analysis of Mobilisation for Youth notes how MFY's community development programme

assisted and strengthened such groups as the Council of Puerto Rican Organisations, consisting of hometown clubs, athletic groups, social clubs, and block associations. Struggling and disorganised, the Council was assigned advisors, the financial resources to set up a headquarters, and other agency services. As a result, it was able to operate a housing clinic, and several of its committees dealt with pubic school problems, police brutality, housing and civil rights. (1969)

A contrast of scale is provided by the example of Cambridge's General Improvement Areas. While relying mainly on resident's committees, which consisted of about fifteen members representing 500 houses, every three months groups of two or three committees came together to discuss points of common interest:

Someone has to collect from the area committees the points they want raised to prepare some sort of agenda in advance of the quarterly meeting. It helps if each area committee has chosen someone to introduce each topic. A newsletter is prepared once a quarter based upon the discussions at the full quarterly meeting. (1978)

We can see how the federated form of organisational structure can have advantages for agencies as well as for the member groups. In the case of Southwark Community Project it became essential to alert local groups to the project's impending withdrawal from the area:

The working party considered a number of options for action after withdrawal, and, in the event, it decided to raise funds in order to employ a community worker and to maintain a locally-managed community work base. The weeks between this decision and the summer of 1972 were full of hard work and anguish for users as they attempted to form themselves into a viable federation of neighbourhood groups. (Thomas, 1976)

There are, accordingly, a range of essentially practical reasons why groups seek to form umbrella organisations. Inevitably, they merge with other motivations of group participants and workers.

Shared Values Between Groups

Building co-ordinating structures for tenants' associations and action groups will take place if groups sense a shared commitment. This can arise when they feel themselves to be under some kind of threat, or when their dissatisfaction, anxiety or anger has reached a similar point. Change of political power, for example, can have the effect of solidifying groups of tenants' associations, particularly when the ruling party's policies, like the selling of council houses and flats, will have drastic effects on council estates. In such situations, creating effective federations of tenants' groups becomes a necessity; they cannot be thought of as simply a more 'sophisticated' form of organising which groups will move towards if and when possible.

If we refer back to the MFY example, Brager and Specht underline the strategic importance of working with strong, inclusive associations:

> From these organisational efforts and effects are forged new political pressure groups. Smaller groups, once voices in an institutional wilderness, are heard – and heeded – as their respective and representative organisations give new voice to their demands. (1969)

In the MFY example there was a direct connection between the practical requirements of weak, separated groups and a strengthening of political resolve, based upon common values. It is a connection which can work in the reverse too: many borough-wide campaigns against racism and fascism in this country have brought together community groups, churches, voluntary organisations, trade unions and others in common cause to combat the manifestation of unacceptable values. In the process, these groupings have sometimes opened up new possibilities of collaboration between groups as well as identified how groups can receive more practical support.

The creation of town-wide or borough-wide organisational structures for groups can emerge slowly, over a period of time, in addition to springing up in response to new situations. It may be that the former are more resilient than the latter. The description by Polanshek (1979) of how residents' committees in Edinburgh's Housing Action Areas came together falls into the category of the gradual development of an additional organising base, from which commonly agreed strategies can be launched.

Structures should arise out of an awareness that (a) groups are tackling similar issues, (b) they frequently have to influence the same target organisations and (c) they will each benefit by capitalising on their common interests by organising together. The work done by a few community projects (Coventry CDP, 1975; North Tyneside CDP, 1978) in making connections between the problems people face in their communities and those they confront at work is based upon the same principles. The two Tyneside CDPs contributed significantly to the North East Trade Union Studies Information Unit.

So far only a small number of neighbourhood workers are making these kinds of links, but as workers acquire more experience of working on the issue of unemployment it is likely that new forms of collaboration between traditionally separate groupings will emerge. It can happen too when factories are threatened with closure or large-scale redundancies: community projects in the north-east have helped to support the formation of inter-union combines, and Coventry CDP was foremost in developing welfare rights services for specific groups of workers who were either being made redundant or were on strike. Bryant's argument for linking community and industrial action requires a lot more testing:

> The failure to relate community work to the economic framework also prevents any systematic consideration of how community and industrial action can be linked, as part of an overall strategy for promoting social change. At the present time in Britain, we find little attention being paid to how community groups may engage in direct forms of economic activity or how relationships might be established between organisations which are active in community and industrial settings. (1974)

Implications of Inter-Group Organising

We have referred already to the two most obvious benefits to be gained by forming umbrella organisations. First, there is increased scope for *co-ordination of activities* of neighbourhood groups which face similar practical problems and which have common interests. The advantages of co-ordination can take various forms. In the Waychester project for example, James, the community worker,

> realised that playschemes could be run more efficiently if resources and equipment were pooled. Instead of a number of independent applications for funds going to the Council and competing against each other, a single application should go in from all the groups. Any errors in the estimates for individual schemes could be corrected by diverting funds from underspent schemes to those in danger of serious overspending. Experience, advertising, equipment and interviewing of playleaders could be shared.

Second, there is the potential for developing a *collective strategy* by groups, and the opportunity to concentrate their resources in campaigns which buttress the work done by groups individually. In this sense an umbrella organisation presents an opportunity for local people to exert more power.

We have juxtaposed two points of origin of umbrella organisations, but for each of them the outcome from that level of organisation appears to be similar. This applies also to other consequences or benefits which flow from decisions of groups to relate to each other in this way. The following are three such consequences which can become evident.

Sharing Facilities or Resources Four or five active groups which agree on effective ways of relating to each other can then often decide to 'come under one roof'. In this way they reduce their individual costs, or acquire a permanent base for the first time. They can also then be in a position to offer facilities such as meeting-rooms and printing facilities to all the community in addition to their existing members. The possibilities of sharing training and educational resources can be another and potentially more significant consequence for groups which share common interests and problems.

Stimulation of New Projects Creation of an additional level of organising can help provide new momentum among active groups, a desire to 'have another go' at a seemingly intractable problem or to tackle something new. For example, a small federation of tenants' associations in one area of south London gave regular support to a new community health project, thereby helping a difficult scheme to make an effective start. There have been examples of flagging but much-needed community newspapers finding a new lease of life following the coalition of community groups, as well as new newspapers covering a wide area being launched. Thus strong umbrella structures can have the effect both of restoring services to the community and of inspiring new schemes.

Establishing New Resources Federations of community groups may decide to pursue new programmes or projects themselves, as opposed to putting their weight behind those of other people; it is worth mentioning, in this context, that the role of umbrella groups in pressing for the setting-up of advice centres and law centres may not be recognised sufficiently. The North Southwark Community Development Group, which included service agencies as well as neighbourhood groups, was successful in obtaining a large grant for five years, to operate a community planning centre. Issues of *Community Action* in recent years suggest a marked increase in borough-wide and city-wide organising, much of it in response to public expenditure cuts, and there is evidence of how such groupings can secure advances and victories which their member organisations would have been unlikely to achieve on their own. There is a useful discussion of tenants' federations in *Community Action* no. 20 (1975).

We end discussion of the federation form of organising by pointing to some of the risks and dangers associated with it. Taylor *et al* (1976) note the crucial importance of timing the formation of a federation correctly. It is essential for a group to be strong in itself before it considers forming serious organisational links with other groups. This must include the availability of individuals who have the skills and time for this kind of work; the problem is that it is often the leaders of local groups who themselves come forward to participate in umbrella organisations, and the consequent burden can become insupportable. The discovery that groups with similar aims operate with very different styles, which may clash in the umbrella situation, is another risk which local groups take. Or the formation of several groups into a federal structure may release latent divisions within a community which thereby becomes collectively weaker in relation to the rest of society. It is also likely that federations are open to manipulation by political parties.

The most serious danger, however, is that the federal focus may have the effect of drawing a group's leaders away from their own group in a major way; ultimately this can lead to a weakening of the group's credibility in the community. 'Losing' leaders in this way is, in effect, another form of co-optation, particularly if the federation begins to assume responsibilities which could be said to lie with the local authority. Leaders begin by learning to be effective at a federal level, but they can end by being able to talk only with each other, or to resource-holders in other organisations. A neighbourhood worker, of course, has an opportunity to point out, when appropriate, that leaders of a community group – chairman, secretary, treasurer – do not necessarily have to be its representatives to other organisations. Yet often it is precisely these individuals who have the energy, interest or ability to take on an additional role.

Finally, we underline the need for federations of community groups, and individuals active within them, to receive adequate support. This may not necessarily always be community work support – strong administrative resources can often be the priority. But frequently such organisations will need to be serviced by community workers, and their role and tasks may acquire a markedly different emphasis than when working directly with community groups. The Waychester project summarised this as 'putting time and energy at the group's disposal, but trying to see that officers carry out the work attached to their positions and ensuring leadership for short periods when no one else is available'.

Constituency and the General Public

The connection between the activities of a community group and the wider community must necessarily be close. In several senses, the community provides the life blood of a group: it is where membership, which is in a continuing state of decline and renewal, comes from. Furthermore, community work values give significant emphasis to the need to ensure that membership of groups is kept as open as possible, and both workers and leaders should try to counteract the tendency of organisations to control who should belong to them.

Second, groups can gain measurable strength by making certain they keep in touch with the wider community. In the final analysis, that will be their constituency. Effective public information techniques by groups (newsletters, public meetings, press statements, etc.) can be used to do this. At the same time, it will be important for groups to listen to what the community is saying about them; this can often be done best through informal channels of communication.

Finally, groups can never afford to forget that their own members form part of a wider community, and they need to be self-critical of the effects that being active with a group can have on their personal and family lives as well as on their relationships with neighbours and friends; for most people the political is inseparable from the personal.

It is essential for community groups to keep a check on how their actions affect the community for less obviously functional reasons too. Dennis (1968) and others, in attempting to disentangle the idea of 'community', have also helped to place the activities of community groups in perspective. Characteristically, only a small proportion of local residents become involved; how the 'silent majority' perceives and passes judgement upon a community group has to concern the latter's members if their work is not to be seen as irrelevant or even alien.

The idea of a group monitoring the effectiveness and acceptability of its work within the community becomes more tangible once it is applied to an analysis of existing power and influence within a community. The cutting edge of organising can frequently only be discerned when it disturbs, or stimulates response from, power-holders or community influentials. Anticipating how they will judge community organising, especially that which relates most obviously to social change objectives, must form a central part of activists' and workers' repertoires.

The significance of this area underlines again the need for workers and groups to have a good understanding of constituencies. If, for example, a worker perceives there to be a tenants' association in existence which is inactive but which retains control of key resources in a community, he cannot consider how to handle that situation without first obtaining a rudimentary understanding of the extent of covert support the association retains in the community, and an assessment of the potential constituency for forming a new tenants' association. In relation to workers' own constituencies, the second Gulbenkian report (1973) refers to the possibility of a worker being 'a potential rival to a councillor', and this has become a well-worn theme in community work.

Yet, while it may be self-evident that workers need to realise that neither they nor the groups with which they work exist in a political vacuum, experience suggests that neighbourhood workers have yet to understand all the implications. It indicates how much more workers can learn and adapt material from the sociology of communities, from studies of local political systems and from recent developments in community politics.

The Social Policy Perspective

The distinction we make between groups which move towards tackling broader issues by allying with each other, and groups which have social policy questions as their central concern, cannot be clear-cut. By the latter we mean essentially a long-term commitment to working on a particular problem which has an obvious national policy dimension. Instances when groups come together simply for tactical reasons, and do not meet again, cannot be said to be working with a social policy perspective.

We shall see that social policy work does not necessarily imply that a group joins with other groups. On the whole, however, it does require a high degree of organisational strength and confidence on the part of community groups. It is possible to identify action by community groups either which is pitched predominantly at a *national* level, or which picks up on social policy issues chiefly at a more *local* level.

We have in mind the situation where a community group or groups decide to take up a national issue, to put time and energy into trying to change legislation or to influence Government policy. Some of the CDPs' approach fitted into this category, the Satley project's work on leasehold legislation (Green, 1975) perhaps being a good example. The determination of a group to

274

press for a test case decision is another expression of a national social policy perspective and here the ruling in 1974 by the High Court of Appeal in favour of the Lower Broughton Housing Action Group in Salford would be an example. The tenants took out summonses against the local authority under the 1936 Public Health Act. The local authority's appeal was dismissed by the High Court.

The work done by the National Consumer Council in helping to form a national federation of tenants' associations illustrates well the national policy potential of community work. While the attempt has met many obstacles, it provides a case study of this dimension. That it stands out as being untypical in British community work, especially when set against the United States experience, should not mean that its potential be underestimated.

When one turns to action on social policy questions by groups at local, city or regional levels, there is considerably more experience upon which to draw. Many groups attempt to give their activities a policy perspective, but there have been a number of campaigns and programmes which stand out as having been especially concerned with national social policies. Three which have commanded attention have been the squatting movement (Bailey, 1973), the opposition to the 1972 Housing Finance Act, and claimants' unions (Jordan, 1973). Squatters have been concerned to expose both the failure of local housing authorities to fulfil their responsibilities and the inadequacies of national housing policies. Opposition to the 1972 Act became manifest in some areas by tenants' groups deciding directly to challege government policy, by campaigning against the Act and by organising rent strikes. Claimants' unions attempt, with varying degrees of success, to challenge the national welfare benefits system through action designed to monitor and challenge the policies of local DHSS offices, They either do this singly or through joint action.

Given community groups' experiences of pursuing a social policy perspective – and we have referred to only a few of them – we need to suggest what definition of social policy we are assuming when we refer to community action which acts upon it. What implications, too, are there for the neighbourhood worker's role when this kind of work is done?

It is often extremely difficult for any practitioner who is absorbed in the details of his or her work, usually in contact with small numbers of individuals in a specific location, to conceive of that work relating to and frequently influencing social policies. The connection to wider processes is hard to make. Neighbourhood workers constitute no exception.

Yet social policies are not formulated within social institutions in isolation from external influences and pressures, and work done by those, as it were, 'at the coal face' can and does have an effect on decision-makers and others who are traditionally classed as having responsibility for policy formulation. It is this interpretation of social policy with which we ally ourselves, and we believe that it is particularly relevant to neighbourhood work. More than most other practitioners, neighbourhood workers have a mandate which encourages them both to 'fill out' social policies, that is, to interpret and discuss them with local people, and also to change social policy.

Workers are right to search for ways of helping the groups with which they work to understand the policy implications of their action. This can range from discussing with a group which is pressing for a community centre the financial and management policies of local and national education authorities to community centres, to sharing with a housing group recent developments in national housing policy; most groups, for example, which advocate improvement of a housing area rather than clearance will need to grasp changes in central government policy at an early stage in their campaign. This example, indeed, is a particularly appropriate one bearing in mind the influence of community action on the shift by government away from wholesale clearance policies towards improvement.

The role of the neighbourhood worker in bringing the policy perspective to community groups' attention is of considerable significance. In terms of having clear ideas and relevant information about social policies, the worker can be an essential resource for a group which is developing its ideas rapidly. The worker can play a supporting role behind a group's turning towards the broader issues which do not relate obviously to a local situation but which in fact can be the determining factors of that situation. The danger to be alert to is that, in a group's involvement with broader policy issues, it does not tend to drift away from its own constituency.

Learning to Administer and Provide Services

Study of the administration and provision of community services touches on a central question in neighbourhood work: to what extent should workers be concerned with helping groups to acquire and provide services, as opposed to facilitating social action and awakening people to opportunities for participating in, and influencing, local decision-making processes and wider social issues? It is easy for both community groups and neighbourhood workers to be drawn increasingly into managing services which they have struggled to obtain:

> I have known workers who have called themselves community workers and have ended up being nothing of the sort. For example a new worker sees a need for youth provision and, rightly thinks something should be done. So he starts running youth clubs or a play project. Very quickly he finds he is just another youth or play leader. Very valuable work, but not, in my estimation, community work. (Twelvetrees, 1974)

We chose to include a section on administering and providing services in this chapter because the questions which it raises are of a similar order to those we have examined in relation to a group's relationship to other systems. Opinion about a potential resource or service will tend to point a group in one direction rather than another. It is therefore useful for a worker to be able to offer some clear thinking on the matter. If a group plans to broaden its work by, for example, joining a tenants' federation, it should be encouraged to think about ways of ensuring the continued strength of its base and avoid overstretching its resources (*Community Action*, 1978).

The difficulty is illustrated by the range of meanings and ambiguities often attached to such phrases as 'self-help' and 'community-based' services. Not everyone, for example, articulates their understanding of such terms as sharply as Heller:

> I would suggest that self-help and community oriented alternatives should be advocated and fought for not because they are cheaper (because they may well not be), or because they require fewer paid staff (because they shouldn't) or because they relieve pressure on statutory services (because pressure is

needed for improvement and many people will always rely on statutory services), but because they are better services. The power of the self-help movement lies in the shift of control over knowledge and the potential for organisation needed to countermand the powerful interest groups, at present in control of the services and manipulating them to their own advantage. (n.d.)

What should accompany a strong value stance like the above are identifiable skills to help people run their own organisations – if that is what they have decided they want to do – so that they have control over what services they wish to offer and how they will provide them. The neighbourhood worker always has to be alert to finding ways of helping groups acquire necessary knowledge and skills to do this. In other words, he has to give explicit recognition to ensuring that needs are met in addition to undertaking the enabling and organising work that so strongly characterises neighbourhood work.

The variety of transactions which occur between local groups and resource-holders suggests, however, that the reality is more complex than a simple flow of resources from those who administer to those who demand them. The work of the Southwark Community Project indicates that there are at least six ways in which community groups attempt to influence resources; and these categories of resource influence are discussed below. They are not offered as a rigid list but as a guide for clearer thinking on this question.

(1) *Resource acquisition*   A local group achieves an increase in, or addition to, a stock of particular resources. The group and its constituency acquire resources to which it has had little or no access. The acquisition of new housing by a tenants' association is an example.

(2) *Resource improvement*   Groups make an improvement in the quality of existing resources and services. For instance, caretaking facilities, transforming static into adventure playgrounds, making officials more responsive to community needs.

(3) *Resource rejection*   A group opposes and rejects the proposed introduction of resources to its community. An example is the

work of the North Southwark Community Development Group in its attempts to keep hotel, office and luxury flat development out of its community. Examples are provided from other areas by airport and motorway opposition groups. The category also includes resisting the perpetuation of unwanted resources in the community.

(4) *Resource conservation* Groups attempt to conserve existing resources in the face of a threat to remove or reduce them. Thus one group may want to conserve a historic building or an open space while another may wish to conserve the real incomes of its members in the face of impending rent increases or reductions in welfare benefits. Community groups who help constituents to resist evictions or harassment by landlords who wish to use the property for other purposes are engaged in the conservation of a housing resource.

(5) *Resource administration* Local residents take on responsibility for administering and managing a local resource (such as a playground, or short-life housing) but where the resources are owned and/or financed by, for instance, the local authority.

(6) *Resource provision (self-help)* Residents attempt to provide services outside and independently of the formal structure of service provision.

The boundaries of these transactions are not always certain or clear, and there may be difficulty in deciding in which category a transaction is to be placed. For instance, the efforts of a tenants' association to achieve rehousing for its constituents may be seen either as resource rejection or, if we look at it from the perspective of the tenants, as resource acquisition (new homes). Likewise, the efforts of parents to open and manage a playground may be seen as both resource acquisition and resource administration. Again, success in modifying the views of officials in the local offices of the Department of Health and Social Security in regard to stigmatised groups (resource improvement) may lead to greater use of discretionary powers and hence to increased welfare benefits (resource acquisition). These examples indicate the difficulties of classification. In some instances different types of resource transaction are different sides of the same coin. Over time the same community groups might fall into different categories, and a number of the classifications are interrelated at any one time or over time.

This conceptualisation of neighbourhood work activities offers a relatively concrete and specific way of ordering an often bewildering diversity of activities. Within each category of resource influence, these activities are seen to have features held in common throughout the fields in which community groups traditionally operate. The categorisation also helps us to see that in any one of these fields community groups are attempting to influence decisions about resources in a variety of ways.

There are an increasing number of case studies which portray the categories of administrating and providing services. The evaluation by Cumbria CDP of the community resource centre in Cleator Moor, and the local management structures set up for it, is a good example. There will be overlap between the activities of the two types of resource management. They each imply, however, differing roles to be played by members of community groups, and by neighbourhood workers. Which type a group should decide to choose must be determined chiefly by particular circumstances; both can involve groups in assuming major responsibilities. Yet a decision of a group to move towards providing services itself usually requires of a group that it is at a more advanced stage of organisational development than a group which undertakes administration of a resource. The former also assumes that, within the group, there are individuals with considerable imagination, experience, skills and perseverance to launch a viable self-help scheme.

It can be argued that service provision has the advantage of being more acceptable to groups than schemes which are acting on behalf of, or with the authority of, another agency. There is always a risk that arrangements made within the second category will deteriorate into a situation where a group is merely subcontracted by the responsible agency, with a consequent disproportionate share of the responsibilities and insufficient benefits. The difference can be illustrated by contrasting a tenants' management scheme and a tenants' co-operative. In the former, tenants are given the responsibility by their landlord to organise the running of their estate or block. In the latter, tenants are involved in the management of their housing as full participants – at least they should be: Crossley and his colleagues subtitle their discussion of tenant co-ops 'Government con trick or a force for tenant power?' (1977). The advantages and disadvantages of the two types of resource management is another debate which a worker can help to draw to the attention of a group.

What can we learn from experiences of the categories of administering services and providing them? We identify four areas:

mutual benefits;
human resources;
workers employed by community groups;
worker role and problems.

Mutual Benefits   Dealings between an action group and its target over resource administration and provision may be effected through collaboration because they are transactions that often carry benefits for the target. For example, a local authority requires management and administrative resources when residents take on responsibilities for managing a playground and employing play leaders, while residents acquire new organising experience in addition to more control over local resources. This mutuality of benefits is often overlooked or thought unimportant as agencies struggle to respond to the change proposals of community groups. Agencies can be aware of negative factors like hostile exposure by the media, irritated councillors and inter-agency tensions. Their attention often needs to be drawn to advantages which accrue to them as a result of community organising, and this can be most evident when groups are administering or providing services.

Human Resources   Different people may be better suited to some kinds of transactions than to others. For instance, residents who work effectively in a community group concerned with resource improvement or administration may not work as effectively with transactions about resource acquisition and vice versa; many local residents who fight to acquire a playground site will not be as interested and effective in administering a play project. This is not to deny the motivation and capacity of local people to change and develop, through learning new skills. We are talking about a gradation of effectiveness, not a rigid categorisation. Many local people have gained enormously from helping to run local services, in terms of political awareness and control: mothers who run playgroups and go on to join the women's movement, or advice centre volunteers who become adept at representing individuals at tribunals, for example.

The shift by a group to administration or provision of services also offers an opportunity to counter a tendency for a group to be over-dominated by a few individuals. Organisational structures established for this purpose may not always succeed. The identification of new tasks and responsibilities can represent, as it were, a break with the past and enable new leaders to come forward.

The injection of new blood into the active leadership of a group may sometimes require open challenge to be made to the existing leadership if it is seen to be ineffective, autocratic or is simply considered to have 'held the reins' of power and authority for too long. There may be conflict here between the qualities and predispositions of individuals who come forward to engage in service provision or administration and the qualities and personality needed to challenge entrenched leadership. We suggest that this is because the former is a less controversial area than, for example, struggles to acquire or reject resources, and it may therefore attract people who lack sufficient will or ability to question the position of established leaders.

Workers Employed by Community Groups   The number of full-time neighbourhood workers in Britain employed by community groups is not insignificant. When we include adventure playground workers, playgroup leaders, information and advice workers and other specialised staff hired by a group to provide a particular service, the topic assumes greater importance. Clearly it speaks directly to values in neighbourhoods about control over decision-making and resource allocation, as well as about employment of local people (Huber and McCartney, 1980) and the 'anti-professionalisation' theme in community work.

There are the inevitable administrative tasks for a group which face any employer: payment of salary, arranging tax, insurance and pensions, and so on. It is essential for a group to have an able, experienced and trusted person who can be responsible for this work, and there should be an awareness by the group of its seriousness. 'Moonlight flitting' by treasurers of groups occurs rarely, but there have been bad experiences where administrative jobs have not been maintained, or where communication between a full-time worker and his or her 'paymaster' has broken down. In the long term, the ability of a group to sustain reliable employment conditions for a worker is as good a test as any of its capacity to run a service.

Careful thinking by a group of the support networks required by a worker should run parallel to strong administration. Lambert and Pearson, writing about how to set up adventure playgrounds, state: 'If you start with just one paid leader, he (or she) will need a lot of solid support and active help from the committee and other volunteers, both on and off site' (1974). Similar advice applies to most kinds of workers employed by groups.

As a group gives consideration to the question of support for a worker, a range of key topics will emerge: a *support group* for the worker which can offer guidance and advice about details of the worker's programme; the opportunity for the worker to have regular meetings with a *consultant*; ensuring that attention is given by the group and the worker to the latter's *training* needs and aspirations; encouraging the worker to meet those doing similar jobs across a wider area than the neighbourhood where he or she is based. Such meetings could either provide additional stimulus and support or be a forum for debate and joint action on common issues. Here we have only listed key areas to be considered by a group concerned to offer effective support to a worker. Despite the work involved in establishing them, any community group which wishes to keep its staff and run an effective service will need to address itself to them as thoroughly as any other agency should do.

Finally, we draw attention to a critical area for workers employed by community groups. Broadly, this turns upon the maintenance of political compatibility between a worker and his or her employer. The classic question of worker accountability is usually debated in the context of a worker and a large bureaucratic organisation, most often a local authority. In one sense the question becomes redundant when a worker is employed by a group – there is no other body to which the worker could be accountable. It would be more accurate, however, to argue that the question has to be reinterpreted in the situation we are discussing. Tension between a worker and his employer can arise over disagreement about either strategies, objectives and methods, or about values and ideology. Even when employed by a group the worker may feel he has accountability to other groups, or to people who are not organised.

Worker Role and Problems   There is little doubt that the area of administering and providing services draws upon a different range of skills on the part of a neighbourhood worker to those he or she uses in most other situations. The advantages of a project or an agency having a clear idea of the knowledge and skills it wants from a worker become apparent here. It can be unrealistic to expect one person to work with groups engaged in a wide variety of resource transactions:

> Community workers who have experience and skills in resource acquisition and rejection may have neither the interest nor expertise to offer to groups concerned with transactions about resource improvement or administration. (Thomas, 1976)

A project which can employ a team of workers is at an advantage, for tasks can be shared among staff according to their abilities and interests. There can be wisdom in rotating some tasks directly to do with service provision. This can avoid a situation developing where one worker becomes trapped into helping to provide a service, such as a resource centre, because local people are not yet able to run it themselves. Changing the full-time worker can prevent one worker from becoming frustrated and can also indicate to sponsors and local people involved that reliance upon a full-time worker cannot continue for ever.

Yet many workers are not members of a neighbourhood work team, and our discussion in this chapter of both how a group relates to the rest of the community and of the topic of service administration and provision illustrates again how workers need to be able to move easily between roles during different phases of the neighbourhood work process. This receives further emphasis from our analysis of endings in neighbourhood work in the next chapter.

CHAPTER 10

Leavings and Endings

The closing phase of the neighbourhood work process is often one of apprehension and difficulty for both workers and group members; yet a search of the literature for advice and understanding about this phase will be rewarded only meagrely. Little has been written by or for neighbourhood workers about the various forms of ending. There is also a dearth of material in related fields such as group work, casework and adult education, though what has been written about endings in group work is relevant to the neighbourhood worker (see, for instance, Northern, 1969; Garland *et al.*, 1972; Hartford, 1971; and, best of all, Heap, 1985).

Endings may *seem* less important and demanding (that is, until the worker is experiencing one!) than the other stages of neighbourhood work such as making contact with local people, and helping them form and run a community group. These earlier phases may be viewed as substantial parts of the work while endings *seem* to be something that occur after the action and are, by implication, therefore less important. This is, of course, untrue because some endings occur during the earlier phases of the work when, for example, the worker decides to leave or a group falls apart. Another reason why theorists and practitioners may give less attention to endings is that endings are bound up with a

285

number of intense feelings experienced by the worker and the group members – feelings of loss, separation, grief and guilt. Endings, too, are inextricably connected to the beginnings of other things: workers and members invariably end in order to begin somewhere or something else, and the feelings about, and demands of, a new situation will probably be sufficiently strong to overcome the outgoing worker's resolve to 'write up' the ending of her work.

The inability to deal adequately with the problem of endings may also be understood by the strong wish, even fantasy, among many in community work to be able to see action in the community as something that has no ending. The Biddles, for example, see community work as a 'non-terminal' continuing process; and one can discern in Alinsky's thinking the idea of the steady growth of a group that links up with a wider social movement, through networks of people's organisations. Those who stress process, educational and political learning goals in community work often seem to believe that individuals and groups move on from task to task, reaching higher and more general levels of understanding and influence. The fact that this rarely happens does not seem to diminish the wish that it *should* happen, and it may be the strength of this wish for permanent activisim that distracts attention from managing endings.

Leavings and endings are also linked to failure. It is of interest that the phrase about ending that is most common in community work – 'the job of the community worker is to put herself out of a job' – assumes success on the part of the worker and local residents. But endings are as often brought about by *lack* of success and progress, either on the part of the worker or of the group. Failure, and the endings associated with it, is something difficult to contemplate particularly among the members of a relatively recent, innovating occupation like community work.

Endings that are brought about by the withdrawal or departure of the neighbourhood worker may be facilitated where the worker has managed to keep the dependency of the group on himself at a fairly low level. The more dependent a group has become on a worker, the harder it will be to manage the worker's leaving and its own affairs after his departure. One of the core skills in neighbourhood work is to provide support, help and resources to a group without this fostering an overdependence of the group on the worker. Yet the need to keep dependence at a low level strains against the equally important need for the worker to 'get close to the group'. Most neighbourhood workers may be seen as outsiders in the communities they work in, by virtue of their class, background, education, life-style and ambitions. Thus most workers have purposefully to build up their relationships with local people, and to communicate their identification with them. It is no easy task both to get close to a group, provide it with support and help and at the same time to foster its independence.

A Comment on Evaluation

The matter of evaluation, to which we shall refer several times in this chapter, is a major topic in its own right. It is impossible within the confines of this book to provide more than a reference to its position within the process of neighbourhood work, and a confirmation of the political and technical difficulties that surround it.

Attempts at evaluation seek to monitor the activities of a neighbourhood work intervention, and to assess the outcomes of such interventions. These outcomes may be either the process or the products of the neighbourhood action. The limitations of classical research designs in community work have been fully discussed in the excellent report by Key *et al.* (1976), which is the best treatment to date in the community work literature of alternative approaches to evaluation. They have developed their work in a further paper (Armstrong and Key, 1979).

In the United States evaluation in community work, social work and social action programmes has been extensively written about. In Britain little evaluation research has been done in community work or related fields. Moseley came to the opinion that 'people working in the field of community development place little value upon formal evaluative research, and show in their writing little awareness of the thought habits which its practice encourages' (1971). An article by Epstein *et al.* (1973) is one of the few British journal references to evaluation in community work, and its United States authors pose four major dilemmas in evaluation: what kind of evaluation? evaluation for whom? evaluation by whom? and evaluation at what cost?

No doubt the methodological problems have deterred many

practitioners from evaluating their work. In addition, neither sponsors nor agencies seem to have accorded much importance to evaluation; the climate in which community work has developed has been relatively free of expectations that evaluation was a likely or desirable outcome to community work initiatives. This attitude may have been influenced by the experience in the United States where programme evaluation 'seems to have relatively little to do with initiating, implementing and modifying service programs' (Meld, 1974). Meld suggests that one reason for this is that evaluation is taken notice of only in the right socio-political climate. As well as this, evaluation research lacks the ability to affect decisions because too many people and agencies acquire vested interests in the continuation of services and projects. A much fuller review of research and evaluation in community work has been provided by Thomas (1980).

It is possible to see that evaluation in neighbourhood work is concerned with four interrelated issues: effects, process, performance and needs.

Effects

We want to know what have been the effects or outcomes of interventions, and to what extent, if at all, they were due to the inputs of the community worker. Knowledge is also desirable on whether the effects were in the direction and with the intensity and quality that were wanted. Other questions are: were there secondary effects? were some effects harmful? how long will the effects persist? were the achieved effects worth the cost of the community work initiative? could they have been achieved in other ways? The methodological problems in getting satisfactory responses to these matters are complex, and especially in the area of assessing process or educational effects – what is a satisfactory index or measurement of 'civic competence', 'political awareness' or 'personal self-confidence'?

Process

Regardless of the effects of what the neighbourhood worker did, it is reasonable to ask what knowledge has been gained about the process of doing neighbourhood work; and to see what has been learnt about the community work agency, other organisations and community residents involved in the piece of action.

Performance

Evaluation here raises questions about the performance of the neighbourhood worker. Did he work hard enough? Did he work in accordance with team and agency policies? How is the *quality* of what he did assessed? What did he, and others, learn about the usefulness of his knowledge and skills as a worker? Were there dysfunctional aspects of what he did that could reasonably have been avoided? Did the piece of work provide clues as to his strengths and weaknesses as a worker?

Needs

Evaluation is often seen as essential because through it workers and agencies can discover new areas of need in the neighbourhood. It is not just that a piece of work may well generate further issues but also the fact that it is through involvement with residents on a particular task that a worker may become better placed to 'see' further needs that were previously hidden to him.

It may be that, with the other tasks associated with ending, most workers would have time for only a cursory attempt at evaluation; there are a number of examples of 'soft-line' evaluation in community projects that can help in this work. For example, there are three books (published in 1976): Jacobs, Thomas and Taylor *et al.*, and that of the Bryants (1982). These are soft approaches because the authors attempt a highly impressionistic evaluation of their work through (a) trying to weigh the relative costs and benefits of their interventions and/or (b) developing a case study of their work and allowing, and sometimes inviting, the reader to make his own assessment of the work.

Whatever the scope and methods of any piece of evaluation in neighbourhood work, its results should never be hoarded by agencies and professionals, Workers must think about the best ways of feeding back evaluative outcomes to neighbourhood groups. Such a process may also help in some of the tasks described in this chapter, such as that of helping residents come to their own evaluation of both their efforts and those of the neighbourhood worker.

Types of Endings in Neighbourhood Work

Endings in neighbourhood work occur in a variety of ways, and we propose to analyse them according to whether they happen to the group or are initiated by the worker.

The Group Comes to an End

A common type of planned ending occurs when a community group accomplishes its goals. In some cases, this will mean the physical breaking-up of the group that has sought rehousing for its constituents, and Thomas has briefly discussed the ending phase of such a group (1975a). More common, perhaps, is the case where a group achieves its goals (or on the other hand recognises that they cannot be achieved), and the members decide it is more appropriate to dissolve the group than to work at new issues. However, its members may remain informally in touch with one another and some may also join other community groups or come together at a later stage to take action on some neighbourhood issue as members of a newly formed group.

A group may also come to an end, first, because it has decided to amalgamate with another group with, say, similar aims and constituents (e.g. the amalgamation of two neighbouring tenants' associations, or that of two pressure groups) and, second, because it has run out of the finance necessary to continue its operations.

Another kind of ending for a group (though it is not strictly an ending) occurs when a group makes a significant *transition* in the nature of its activities. Transitions of this kind have to be prepared for and managed by worker and group as diligently as real endings, and should involve *rites de passage* that formally recognise and facilitate the transition experienced by the group. There are a number of such transitions in community work. For example, a group that has succeeded in *acquiring* a new resource in the neighbourhood like a youth club has to face the transition to *managing* the resource and, as we discussed in the last chapter, this will make different demands on the time, knowledge and skills of its members. A group that has achieved its objectives may decide to stay together and pursue a new set of goals that relate to a 'new' need in the area that perhaps its previous work has unearthed. And a group may decide to work solely through a larger federated organisation of community groups. This is the kind of 'larger nucleus group' identified by the Biddles through which a smaller group makes the transition necessary for dealing with wider community, city and regional issues. This matter was discussed in Chapter 9.

So far we have identified a number of ways in which endings in neighbourhood work occur in a planned manner. Naturally, the corollary of an ending that is planned to take place is that both worker and group will have to deal with feelings and emotions about the ending, and carry out tasks that prepare for that ending and its consequences. In the later part of this chapter we shall look more closely at these feelings and tasks. While many of them are generic to the different types of planned endings that we have discussed, it is also true that each type of ending will make different demands on the worker and the group.

But endings also occur unexpectedly. By their nature, unplanned endings almost always constitute, or revolve around, a crisis in the life and work of a community group. The premature ending of a group may come as a shock and surprise to its members, but the factors that lead up to and bring about such endings may often be discerned by members and worker in advance of the ending. Sometimes group and worker can cope with events so as to avert or postpone the ending; at other times, group and worker feel powerless to intervene to arrest the dissolution of the group.

There seem to be three kinds of developments through which unplanned endings occur.

(1) There is a sudden and extensive loss of the group members or its leaders. Such a loss may occur in a variety of ways, including mass resignation of officers and key members, the withdrawal of support by the group's constituency, and the failure of an annual meeting to elect a new committee. Additionally, groups in which officers have carried the burden of the work may break up if those officers suddenly are unable to carry out their duties because, for example, of illness, arrest by the police or rehousing. Conflicts between members are an

ever-present possibility of group life and can lead to splits within a group and its collapse.

(2) There is a gradual loss of membership and the group withers away despite the work of some group members and the worker to reinvigorate the group and attract new members. Gradual loss of membership may occur because of apathy, slow progress, and lack of interest in the issue pursued by the group. Also, people may become deterred from remaining or becoming members of a group if they believe that to do so would jeopardise their interests.

(3) There is a crisis in the group precipitated by the death or serious illness of a key person.

Unplanned endings such as these pose particular problems for the worker, not least feelings of guilt that the events that led to the endings might have been averted or foreseen if the worker had been more skilled, or less harassed by demand from other groups and from his agency. The worker has to decide whether to put time and energy into starting the group again, or whether it would be better for him to move on to some other issue or group. If he believes it is right to help to start the group again, and he is encouraged to do so by local people, he then has to face, together with the rump of local people who remain, other decisions about the goals, activities and procedures of the re-formed organisation.

The prospect and the actuality of the ending of a community group are likely to cause a variety of emotions and feelings in the group members. The reason for the ending of a group will naturally determine the kinds of ways in which the members experience ending. The premature ending in crisis, and without much to show for its work, of a group, is likely to leave its members disillusioned, with feelings of failure and a wariness of collective action that may make them reluctant to join a community group ever again. On the other hand, the ending of a group that has successfully achieved its goals will leave its members strengthened and confirmed both in their personal abilities and in the efficacy of collective action.

Even when the work of a group comes to a successful conclusion, the feelings of achievement of its members will be tempered, and may be over-ridden, by feelings of uncertainty and loss – loss of the support and friendship found in the group, and loss of the opportunities for creativity, helping others, responsibility, authority and status that were present in the work of the group. For many members, the group will have had a major impact on their lives, affecting their family and work, and many will ask the question, 'what now?'. If the work of the group becomes less and less demanding as ending approaches, members may encounter the kind of emptiness in their lives that they fear when the group eventually breaks up. Thus the prospect of ending will provoke a welter of ambivalent feelings amongst the members and, as we shall discuss later, it is the task of the worker to help the group 'work' on these feelings and understand the kind of effect they may be having on the day-to-day business of the group.

The Neighbourhood Worker Decides to Leave

The decision of the worker to end or reduce his association with a community group is the occasion for quite a different type of ending. There are a number of ways in which this can occur.

The worker decides to change his job and move to another This invariably but not always involves the worker leaving his agency and ceasing to work in the area in which the community groups he has worked with are located. There are diverse reasons why a worker will move on to another job, including the desire for change, better work prospects and a more congenial agency setting. In some cases, a worker may decide to leave an agency as a result of a disagreement with his supervisors about the activities of a group, and his relationship to it. There are various possibilities through which a group and the outgoing worker can manage this situation.

(1) The outgoing worker seeks to hand over his work to his successor and, with the consent of the group(s), introduces his successor to the people he has been working with. Adequate record-keeping is essential in facilitating an effective hand-over of work. The worker may also promote with the group and his agency the suggestion that local people are involved in the selection of his successor. The *way* in which the incoming worker is introduced to the local groups can be a major determinant of his future relationship with them. The different levels of care and attention that a new worker may experience in being introduced is

captured in the following extract from a new worker's records at the Southwark Community Project:

> With Ogden House, I developed a relationship with individual committee members before attending my first meeting. This was especially the case with the Chairman who took it upon himself to introduce me to the project patch as well as to the Ogden House situation. With Leighton Street playground, however, I was catapulted straight into a committee meeting without first having had the chance to meet individual members. The difficulties caused were compounded by the fact that Joan [the outgoing worker] came late for the meeting and I was not introduced to anyone until the meeting had finished. I then experienced considerable difficulties in getting to talk with the Chairman, though I did easily manage to meet other committee members before the next meeting.

There is value in both the new and outgoing worker holding joint sessions with the local people with whom they work because if the old worker enjoys a good relationship with the group he can help legitimate the new worker.

(2) The outgoing worker hands over his responsibilities to a local person, who has been 'trained' and prepared in anticipation of the worker's departure. This indigenous worker may be an unpaid local activist or a resident employed by a local group(s) that has managed to raise money to hire a community worker.

(3) A local agency or institution like a settlement house undertakes to support the group.

(4) The group joins a federation or coalition of other community groups.

(5) The group decides to carry on without another worker, and without seeking help from local agencies, though it may use them for specific resources and information.

Each of these arrangements for carrying on after the worker's departure has its own costs and benefits, and these need to be assessed in the light of the particular needs and circumstances of each group.

(1) *Finance for the worker's activities comes to an end or, in some cases, is withdrawn.* This situation is 'built in' to those community work projects that come into a neighbourhood for a fixed period, usually three or five years. As we shall discuss later,

part of the worker's tasks may be to help the group(s) to raise money to employ their own staff.

(2) *The worker remains in her job, agency and neighbourhood but believes that the time has come to end or reduce her activities with a particular group.* The worker may reach this decision because she believes other groups in the neighbourhood are in greater need of the services she offers, or because she believes that the group is now able to function either without her help or with her involvement reduced so that she becomes merely someone who provides specific resources and information. The worker may decide either that the group no longer needs the kind of contribution she has been making, or that if it does it can either provide it from amongst its own members or seek it from other people in the area, either local people or other professionals.

This kind of withdrawal by the worker from an ongoing group may be handled in one of two ways. First, there is the time-centred approach in which the worker has made it clear from the first contact with the group that she will be withdrawing after a certain time such as eighteen months or two years, though she indicates she will be flexible about the exact timing of the withdrawal. The advantages of this method are that the reality of the worker's leaving is always clear to the group and that it may increase their motivation to achieve their goals before the worker leaves. Such a contract about withdrawal can also include the possibility of a worker saying she will *partially* withdraw at the end of a time-period, and be available thereafter on a consultancy basis.

The second approach is more goal-centred and has two variations. In the first, the worker makes it clear to the group from the start that she will withdraw when the group has achieved certain goals. These goals may be agreed upon by worker and group. The advantage of this variation is that it appears less arbitrary than using time to determine withdrawal, and the worker leaves the group when its morale and confidence should be high as a result of achieving its goals. A possible drawback of this approach is that the group may 'put off' attaining its goals in order to hang on to the worker; also, it may not be possible to achieve agreement between the worker and the group about whether or not the goals have been achieved.

The second variation of this goal-centred approach occurs when the worker comes to a decision that the goals have been reached, or that the group is well on the way to achieving them. The worker's assessment of the group's progress, and her decision to withdraw, are, so to speak, sprung upon the group – there was no contract or understanding from the outset of the action that the worker would make such an assessment and consider her withdrawal. The worker's decision may be made public, in which case she informs the group of the decision to withdraw, or private, in which case she assesses the group's progress and begins gradually to drift away from it, becoming less and less involved in its activities. Clearly, a disadvantage of this second variation of the goal-centred approach is that the worker's 'sudden' announcement of her withdrawal may affect the group's progress towards the goals in question. And no matter how well the worker explains her decision and reasoning behind it, there is a good chance that her motivations will not be fully understood by the group who may be left feeling let down and rejected.

Whichever approach the worker uses – time- or goal-centred – he will feel uncertain and apprehensive about the rightness of the decision, and the validity of the criteria used in setting the time and goal boundaries. No matter how confident the worker is in the autonomy and resources of the group, he will still worry about whether the group 'can manage without me'. In particular, he will be aware of limitations that exist on the autonomy of the group, including those mentioned by Taylor *et al.* (1976): residents take part in community groups in their spare hours, with limited time and energy at their disposal. They may be unlikely to develop the knowledge, and skills, resources and contacts, of a full-time worker, and they will not have access to the kinds of resources that a worker may exploit in his own agency. The outgoing worker will also wonder about the group's strengths in being able to deal with conflicts and problems arising within the group – disagreements and rivalry, for instance, abut policy, money and leadership. Though worker and group may be confident about how the group has learnt to tackle issues and deal with problems in the past, they may be less certain about the group's ability to generalise what has been learnt and to apply such learning to new situations that arise in the future. In addition, both worker and group may be apprehensive about how well the group will identify the resources it needs to carry out its tasks, and how able it will be in acquiring those resources.

The group that faces the prospect of losing its neighbourhood worker will experience a range of feelings, including, again, a sense of loss. A group, too, may feel guilty – believing it made too many demands on the worker, or that he lost patience with it. There may possibly be a sense of failure if the members think that the worker's departure signals a lack of faith and confidence in them. It is important to note that such feelings and fantasies about losing a worker may characterise even the most independent and successful of groups. If the worker stays on in the neighbourhood to help other groups, some members of the group from which he is withdrawing will feel slighted, unimportant, rejected and envious of the other groups with whom the worker will be in contact.

Apprehensions about the future may also appear in the group as the day for the worker's withdrawal approaches. Members will privately and publicly voice their fears that without the worker they will not be able to deal with the problems that will crop up in their work. Indeed, in the last period of association with the group the worker can expect to encounter two phenomena that may be seen as unconscious 'ploys' to persuade him from leaving. The first is a series of crises in the life and work of the group – about, for example, leadership bids or money – that are 'designed' to show the worker that the group is not ready to function without him; and second, officers will 'contrive' to carry out the tasks of the group with less confidence and skill than characterised their work in the past in order to demonstrate their felt inability to carry on the leadership of the group without the support and advice of the worker. Needless to say, these negative feelings and fears will coexist with feelings of achievement and mastery, and of independence of the worker.

The Experience of Endings

There are a number of ways in which groups manage their feelings about the ending of a group, or the withdrawal of a worker. Reviewing research into behaviour in groups facing ending, Hartford has written that there occurs

an upsurge of clinging together, getting to work more

enthusiastically on the group task, rejecting the work of the group altogether, rejecting leadership, projecting group faults and failures on the group leadership or staff, individual depression, lowering of group morale, abdication of responsibility, excessive absenteeism, [and] regression to previous dates of group disorganisation. (1971)

Our own experience suggests that conflict between committee and constituency, and disputes within the committee about the behaviour and decisions of the officers, are common behaviours in community groups facing termination. There occurs, too, a denial of the impending reality of the ending and groups will try to 'postpone' the ending by:

(1) becoming inefficient in their business through absenteeism; lateness; forgetting to bring papers to meetings and to follow up on decisions made at meetings; and becoming more lax about decisions about the time, place and purposes of meetings;
(2) looking around for other issues and problems to take up, no matter how inappropriate;
(3) becoming reluctant to carry out and complete their tasks;
(4) moving into being friendship and solidarity groups.

Some members may find their anxieties about ending are so hard to bear that they unconsciously want to 'end' before the end of the group. They will perhaps cease to attend meetings and behave to all intents and purposes as if the group's work were complete, or become involved in disputes in the group that threaten to accelerate its termination. This may go hand in hand with attempts to disparage the work of the group and to refuse to acknowledge both what individual members gained from the group and its success in achieving its goals.

We conclude this section by summarising the kinds of reaction to termination that Garland and his colleagues stated 'have been observed repeatedly in groups which were in the process of termination. They are devices typically employed by members to avoid and forestall terminating, on the one hand, and to face and accomplish it, on the other' (1972). The six basic reactions are:

Denial This is achieved in two ways. First, members may 'forget' about termination, and appear surprised when the worker draws their attention to it. Second, members deny termination by 'clustering' together to form a 'super-cohesive' group. This super-cohesiveness is facilitated in community groups because they can scapegoat the authorities with whom they have been negotiating.

Regression Members backslide in their ability to deal with interpersonal and organisational tasks. Disagreements and quarrels may erupt, particularly directed against the leadership and the worker. The group may also revert to levels of functioning that were characteristics of its earlier days.

Clinging The members will deal ineffectually with the group's business, or bring up new problems for the group, because there will be a feeling that the worker will stay on, or the group will continue, if the members can demonstrate the need.

Recapitulation The group will throw up demands to review and even repeat experiences and events that occurred in its formative days.

Evaluation Recapitulation, particularly through review sessions, may lead the group into discussing the value of the group's work and the experience of the group by individual members.

Flight There are two kinds of flight. The first is a 'destructive reaction to separation' in which the members will deny any positive experiences gained in and from the group. The second form of flight is more constructive and members attempt to 'wean' themselves from the group by developing contacts and interests outside the group. 'The new contacts, which may be started well in advance of termination, serve to substitute for interests and gratifications which will no longer be fulfilled after the group's end. They also represent a broadening and maturing of interests and skills'.

So far we have discussed some of the kinds of ways in which group members may experience endings. We now turn to look at the feelings of the neighbourhood worker. He, too, is likely to have made close and satisfying relationships with people in the group, and in its constituency. He will have invested his skills, energy and time into helping the group form, develop and achieve its objectives. He will have struggled with the group through periods of decline, low morale and conflict when the possibility of achieving anything may have looked remote. It is not surprising, therefore, that a worker facing the end of a group or his own withdrawal will also experience some feelings of loss, as well as those of pleasure in noting the progress of the group toward independence and goal achievement. The days before termination/ withdrawal are, for the neighbourhood worker, a period in which he will reflect upon, and evaluate, his contribution to the work of the community group, analysing and learning from the good and bad aspects of his interventions. This kind of self-evaluation is likely to be linked to the worker's attempts to anticipate the kind of challenges he will face in his next job.

The worker may feel anxious about the quality of his work with the group, and inevitably he will feel that he could have done more. The events in his work that he sees as failures will loom large, perhaps overshadowing that which he has done well and conscientiously. His worries about the quality of his work may be exacerbated if he falls prey to assimilating the group members' own sense of failure and disparagement which, we have noted, may characterise their feelings as the termination date approaches. The worker who is leaving for another job may also experience some guilt if he is looking forward to leaving, and if he is leaving in order to go to a 'better job' with more pay and responsibility. He may wonder whether his own self-advancement is being achieved at the expense of the progress of the community group.

The worker who is withdrawing from, or reducing her services to, a group in order to work with others in the area may be apprehensive about the rightness of her assessment of the group's competence. She will want to be sure that her reasons for withdrawing are really what she thinks they are – she must be certain that she is withdrawing because the group no longer needs her contribution and not because she wants to escape from problems and difficulties encountered in working with the group. She must then manage her worries about whether the group will continue to cope without her, and form some confidence that the gains made by the group are relevant and likely to endure in the work it faces in the future.

Finally, we must consider that the worker who is changing her job and leaving the community altogether will be leaving behind far more than the people she has worked with in the particular community group(s). First, she will have feelings about leaving those – probably other professionals – who have worked with her in supporting the neighbourhood group, and she may wonder whether they construe her leaving as a desertion and a lack of commitment to the group and the area. She may feel guilty at leaving them 'to carry the can', and apprehensive about their ability to support the group alone and the effect of their different values and approaches on the work of the group.

Second, the worker will be leaving her colleagues in her agency or community work project. Assuming she is leaving the agency on good terms, she has to manage her sense of loss of colleagues and friends. In particular, her seniors and colleagues are likely to express some remorse that they have not done more in relating to the worker's activities, and in providing adequate support for the worker. It may be that in some agencies the departure of the first neighbourhood worker to be appointed to the staff signals the completion of an innovation or experiment, and staff have to consider whether or not to appoint another worker. This agency assessment of the worker's contribution is yet another aspect of the period of evaluation that occurs in the termination of work.

The Tasks Involved in Endings

It should be clear from the discussion that both the community group and the neighbourhood worker have to carry out certain tasks in order to prepare for, and finally achieve, the ending of the group or the withdrawal of the worker. Ending is a phase in the life of a group or relationship that has to be worked upon just like any of the other phases in group development.

A familiar distinction in the group work literature is that between the phases of pre-termination, termination and post-termination. We shall use these phases (though using different words to describe them) to consider the tasks facing the group and the worker in endings.

Before the Ending Happens

In this phase, there are four tasks to be carried out. They are: evaluation; disengaging from relationships; stabilising the change effort; and administration (Pincus and Minahan, 1973).

Evaluation Here, the task of the neighbourhood worker is twofold. First, she must help the group to evaluate its own experience and achievements, partly in order to help members achieve the kind of recognition and reinforcement of their progress that will promote confidence in themselves when the worker has left, or when the group finishes. Second, the worker must encourage some evaluation by group members of her own contribution to the group. This is done partly to see how far the worker has achieved the goals outlined in her initial agreement with the group, and partly as an aid to the group in planning the resources it will need in the future. Identification of the kind of contribution of the worker will better enable the group to assess if it can now make that input from within its own members, if it is still needed; and what resources it will need that have to be obtained from outside the group. The worker may need to foster such evaluation with individual members of the group and with the group in one of its own committee sessions. Achieving an effective balance between private and public work is one of the skills of carrying out the pre-termination tasks.

Disengaging from Relationships The most important task of the worker is to help the group acknowledge and confront the reality of ending and then to help members openly to discuss their attitudes and feelings. As we have already noted, there may appear in a group a number of behaviours that seek to deny or forestall the fact of termination, and the worker must be able to recognise these and use them to encourage the group members to admit the reality of ending and to prepare for it.

The worker must introduce the subject of ending or withdrawal early enough for the group to work positively on it, but not so soon that people's feelings about termination serve to inhibit the achievement of the group's goals. His purpose in encouraging openness about ending is to ensure that felt but unexpressed emotions do not negatively affect the work of the group in its last period, nor the relationship between people in the group. Again, it is important to note that the worker will probably have to work with individuals and the group in this task of disengaging from relationships with the group. The worker who is leaving a group may be tempted to discuss his leaving only with individual members of the group (and, perhaps, only the officers). But even if all the group members know of his leaving and have discussed it with him, there is every reason to encourage the members to discuss the issue as a group. His leaving is, after all, a group problem, and it is the group that will need to discuss how they will prepare for his leaving and the period afterwards.

The other aspect of the disengagement of relationships is the worker's attempts to reduce his involvement in the affairs of the group. This will typically be the concern of a worker who is withdrawing from the group or who is leaving to take up another job. What the worker has first to accomplish is a willingness in himself to let go; he must then decide upon the speed and timing of his steps to reduce involvement. There are no general prescriptions to help him in this task for he must take into account the particular circumstances of the group he is working with. He must also decide whether his decision to reduce his involvement is a private one, or whether it is one he will share either with a group's officers or with the group as a whole. Again, he must decide this on the basis of his knowledge of the group and the nature of his relationships with its members. Some openness about his interventions may be desirable, however, for group members will inevitably soon perceive the ways in which he is cutting down on his involvement. The risk that the worker runs in concealing his intentions is that group members may misinterpret his reduced involvement as a rejection of themselves, or as a lowering of his commitment to them and their work. Both these perceptions may adversely affect the work of the group.

There are a number of ways in which the neighbourhood worker can detach himself from a group in anticipation of his withdrawal or departure:

(1) reducing the number of committee meetings of the group that he attends;
(2) being present for only part of meetings by arriving late or leaving early; a worker may arbitrarily decide how long to be

at a meeting, or to be present only for some agenda items and not for others;

(3) contributing less and less to discussion during meetings of the group;

(4) absenting himself from the informal, but highly important, meetings of some group members that frequently occur before and after committee meetings;

(5) reducing attendance at meetings that the group holds with other groups and organisations;

(6) deciding not to get to know new members of the group who join in the period before his leaving;

(7) introducing new resources to the group – other professionals or his successor as community worker;

(8) reducing social contacts with group members.

The worker who is housed in an accessible neighbourhood base like a community work project or an advice centre may also decide to stay away from the base for a period each week, say, a day. This absence will help to reduce his availability to group members and facilitate other tasks he has to carry out before his departure, such as the writing up of his records.

Stabilising the Change Effort   The worker's concerns in this task are, according to Pincus and Minahan, those of assessing:

> the steps which must be taken to make sure that the positive changes and gains will be maintained after he is no longer involved . . . the worker must assess what factors may counter-act the change effort and take steps to prevent such an occurrence. (1973)

To help stabilise the change, the neighbourhood worker tries to provide the kind of continuing support the group might need.

The neighbourhood worker seeks to leave the group feeling confirmed in its abilities and reasonably confident about meeting the challenges that lie ahead. This is achieved partly through taking opportunities with group members to assess the work of the group, and explicitly to recognise the progress that has been made by the group and by individuals within it. But chance, too, plays a part in this stabilisation process and the worker might hope in the period before her withdrawal/departure that no real crisis (as opposed to those manufactured by the group to persuade the worker to stay on) or heavy demands will appear to test the group's confidence and perhaps to undermine it.

In addition, there are a number of things that the worker may consider doing to stabilise and strengthen the community group. These may include:

(1) *Working with the group to discuss whether or not it wishes to make use of the services of the worker's successor, if there is to be one.* The group may also want to discuss with the worker whether or not it will be participating with the agency in matters like preparing a job description, interviewing and selection. A community worker in a project that has come to the end of its finance and is closing down might also work with a group, or federation of groups to raise finance and other resources like office space to employ its own staff. If this is successful, then further work must be done with the group in coming to a decision about what kind of staff it wants, the work they will do, and the kind of arrangements that are necessary for advertising, interviewing and selection.

(2) *Ensuring with the group that its structure and procedures are as stable as possible for the tasks that lie ahead.* The group's constitution, and its arrangements for dealing with finance, the election of officers and the recruitment of new members, might be reviewed at this stage.

(3) *Discussing with other outsiders and professionals the nature of their continuing contribution to the group after the worker has left.* The worker must ensure that they relate directly to the group and see the need for remaining available to the group as resources. She must ensure that these other professionals do not see themselves as relating to the group through herself, because if they do their association with the group may fall away after she has gone. Additionally, the worker may discuss with the group what new resources, if any, it will need in the future, and the identification and acquisition of these resources will be part of her work in the pre-termination phase.

Mitton and Morrison in their account of community work in Notting Dale suggest there may be a danger in introducing new resources, particularly new members, in the pre-termination phase (1972). While new members are necessary, it might not be the best time for them to be given responsibilities within the group, for if they fail (through lack of experience and skills, for instance) this might lower morale and confidence in the group at a time when it needs to be as high as possible. The neighbourhood worker perhaps needs to discover whether in the pre-termination phase a group can cope with and tolerate newcomers; if she thinks that it can, she must help the group assimilate and welcome them without giving them too much initial responsibility. The primary task in this phase is, after all, to build upon and consolidate what the existing members have learned and achieved.

(4) *Clarifying with service agencies in the neighbourhood the nature of their continuing relationships, if any, with the group.* This would include indicating to agencies the kinds of resources they have available that might be needed by the group.

(5) *Clarifying the extent to which she, the worker, will be available after the date of her departure/withdrawal;* and agreeing on the kinds of issues which it might be appropriate for the group to bring to the worker. The nature of her availability is a difficult decision for the worker; besides constraints on her time, she will not want to agree to any arrangements that she suspects will foster the dependence of the group on herself. On the other hand, she will not want to give the impression that she does not care about, or is not interested in, the continuing fortunes of the group. Neither will she want to appear to intrude upon the efforts of her successors in establishing relations with the group. At the very least, the worker may want to leave her telephone number, though Mitton and Morrison have warned of the dangers of this; namely, that the telephone number may not be available to new members that join. This could lead to situations in which the worker is being consulted by one faction in a group, and not by the other. Her picture of events is then incomplete.

The worker may also seek to make other kinds of arrangements for keeping in touch with the group; for example, she may ask the group to send her its minutes, newspaper clippings, reports, and so forth, and express her interest in attending group events like fund-raising occasions, social outings and the annual meeting. She may, too, want to remain in touch with other professionals and service agencies in the area who could pass her news and information about the work of the group.

The worker must bear in mind in seeking to clarify the nature of her availability after the group ends that group members will have formed their own views about it. It will be part of her task openly to discuss with people her and their expectations about future contacts. The failure to do so may result later in uncertainty on the part of group members and the worker, and feelings of disappointment, rejection and resentment. Some of the uncertainties about what to do, and the mixture of feelings about keeping up contacts, are captured in the following record of a neighbourhood worker:

> I didn't hear anything from the group for several months, though I did learn that John (the other community worker who had left with me) was paying regular visits to the area. This worried me partly because we had agreed not to do anything that made the groups reliant on us, and partly because I was envious that he and his groups were still working together. Then, I began getting copies of the minutes of the playground committee and invitations to come to its jumble sale etc. There were, too, a few telephone calls from Fred [the chairman of a group] full of news about the group, and saying I should come down for a drink, though we never actually fixed a date. Two people from Burnsville TA also got in touch, one for me to stand bail, and the other for me to act as guarantor in an HP agreement. During this time, I couldn't decide whether to take these cursory contacts at their face value and accept the groups were getting on alright, or whether to see them as signals that some help and advice were needed and that I should take the initiative in finding out what was going on.
>
> After about 18 months of this sporadic contact, things seemed to change. Fred and his two urban aid workers did get around to fixing a few drinks sessions, and even to invite me to their AGM, which I actually had to chair for five minutes whilst the new officers were elected. There seemed to be more openness towards me, and Fred said something about how they thought the time was now ripe for them to have me down and show me how they were getting on. I understood this to mean that they had needed to go through a period in which they demonstrated (to themselves and me) their independence of me and the whole Project set-up which had been in the area for several years. Having done this, they were now ready to

welcome me on a peer basis; there would be no doubts in anybody's mind that they were seeking 'help' or that they were not managing.

(6) *Helping the group develop and consolidate its relationships within the wider community.* This is, of course, particularly important for members of a group that is ending because it has completed its tasks. Members may need support and advice in finding elsewhere the opportunities they found through membership of their group. Particularly important for members may be alternative sources of friendship, support and outlets for creativity and continuing involvement in civic affairs or community action. Likewise, the worker may need to assist an ongoing group to make the contacts with other organisations in the community that might be useful in pushing forward the future work of the group.

Administration The fourth set of tasks for the neighbourhood worker in the pre-termination phase may be seen as basically administrative and relating more to his agency or project than to the group(s) with whom he works. Because the worker is likely to be very busy in the period before he leaves, these agency-based responsibilities may tend to get pushed aside in favour of time put in with group members. There seem to be four important administrative tasks for the worker.

(1) *The writing up of records and the preparation of reports on the work.* The worker will need to complete this writing in order to facilitate the orientation of his successor to the work; to prepare a base from which he and his agency may evaluate the nature of his work; and to guide and influence the agency in their future development of community work. The worker may also want to prepare papers for dissemination or publication that illustrate what he sees as important issues and ideas that have arisen from his work.

(2) *The evaluation of his work with his agency supervisor and colleagues.* Evaluation is important not least because professionals in public service must attempt to assess how effective they have been in achieving their goals, but also because it is a learning experience from which the agency can benefit in the drawing up of proposals for the employment of another community worker to

replace the one who is leaving. The worker should also learn from evaluation things that will be helpful in his future practice, and particularly feed-back from the agency about how he has worked as a colleague and change agent within the agency. The worker, too, can give feed-back to his supervisor and to the agency in general about the nature and quality of the support for his work that he has experienced in the agency. This kind of evaluation is essential if a worker and his agency are to develop in their practice and management of community work.

(3) *Effecting closure on his relationship with agency colleagues and those in other agencies with whom he has worked.* Such closure is too often confined to informal social events, but there is a need to create opportunities for the worker to discuss his work with his colleagues inside and outside the agency. Such discussions might be based upon papers prepared by the worker about the different aspects of his work.

(4) *Clarifying with his agency what is to be done about appointing a successor.* This may involve making the case for the continuation of a neighbourhood work appointment because other staff may press to use the post to employ another type of worker; hence, the effective evaluation of his work will have an important influence on whether the agency continues to employ a neighbourhood worker. The worker might also seek to clarify what role, if any, local groups will play in discussions about appointing a new worker.

The Ending

At the point of termination, the community worker's main task is to ensure that the group gives itself what Baldock has called a 'decent burial'. He writes:

> There is a great danger that people will be left feeling that the experience was not worthwhile, that 'it's useless trying to start anything around here'. It may be valuable for the group to wind up formally with an appreciation of what it has been able to achieve, quite apart from the fact that the existence of funds may make a formal dissolution necessary. But the burial should be a decent one. (1974)

The ending of a group may be formally achieved through a

meeting that makes arrangements about the disposal of funds and what is to be done about dealing with correspondence and other issues that might occur; and through some organised social event like a party or outing that marks the ending of the group. The literature on social group work emphasises the importance for termination of some ritual or closing ceremony that helps members make the final acknowledgement of the ending of the group. It has been suggested that activities that help towards marking the fact of termination should be guided by three major principles: first, they should indicate and confirm the success of the group; secondly, they should be activities and events that reduce the cohesiveness of the group; thirdly, activities should help members to consolidate their attempts to reach outside the group.

Some workers have been embarrassed (but perhaps inwardly pleased) by some of the events arranged by community groups to mark ritually the departure of the worker or the ending of the group. The worker may be formally given a gift at the last meeting, or made the subject of speeches of gratitude at farewell parties.

After the Ending

We have already discussed that the worker and group members may have a variety of social and/or work contacts after the event of a group's ending or a worker's departure or withdrawal. Additionally, the worker may renew contact with group members if she has written up her work and she wants their comments on her drafts. The worker, too, may have some obligation to evaluate her work through obtaining consumer views of this contribution and she (or a researcher) may wish to interview group members and local residents about the community work services they have previously received.

Workers who have moved into teaching posts may want to call upon group members to take part in seminars with the students. Finally, workers may want to contact members in order to obtain a 'community reference' for a new job for which they are applying.

Conclusions

We have endeavoured in this chapter to indicate that leavings and endings have to be thought about and planned for, just like any other phase in the process of doing community work. They must be managed effectively not least because a group member's experience of the ending of a group will be an important influence upon her attitude towards engaging in collective action in the future, or in feeling confident enough to place neighbourhood issues in a broader social and economic context. If first impressions count, last impressions linger, and the neighbourhood worker should do all she can to avoid unhappy endings overshadowing the positive aspects of the group's activities.

CHAPTER 11

A Little More About Process

In this chapter, we want to develop some of the ideas of process, theories and values discussed at the beginning of the book. We will do this by examining in more detail different kinds of propositions in community work. We want to distinguish propositions of practising or doing community work (practice theory) from those that treat community work as an object or phenomenon, in its own right worthy of scrutiny and explanation (know-about propositions).

Practice Theory

These kinds of propositions contribute to a theory of the doing of community work. It is possible, following Kramer and Specht (1975), to see that there are two kinds of propositions that make for the development of a practice theory in community work. They are know-how and know-why propositions.

Know-How Propositions

These suggest the activities and tasks of community work, and often describe them in terms of principles, methods, guidelines and operations. The purpose of these propositions is instructional –

their function is 'to advise how to do'. Their nature, if they are to be used effectively, needs to be as specific and concrete as possible.

These propositions are an answer to the question 'what *do* community workers *do?*'. They are not necessarily written in the style of a manual or a cookbook; rather they specify the range and sequence of operations in community work, and the tasks the worker needs to do in order to accomplish the operations. For example, one level of know-how proposition would describe the activities of the worker in 'providing information and resources'. More specific propositions would then follow about what the worker *does* in providing information and resources – his or her role, methods, presentation, relationships with information providers and users, and so on.

There are a variety of ways in which people wanting to learn to do community work absorb and analyse know-how propositions. They are the object of learning in field placements, apprenticeships and skill-development in workshops that use video. Such propositions are also implicit in case studies of practice, or in accounts of community work projects. They are very often explicit in papers and books that deal with topics such as role, tactics and strategies in community work; and are the backbone of papers that treat matters such as 'how to get into the neighbourhood' or 'how to use video in community work'.

One of the difficulties facing the learner in assimilating know-how propositions is that of finding order and sequence in the variety of tasks that we will find enumerated in the literature and revealed in field practice. One of the ways of providing this order is to define a number of skill areas in community work. Bryant and Holmes (1977), for instance, refer to engagement, organisational, planning and policy, action, communication and political skills.

As we suggested in Chapter 1, one means of achieving this order is in the notion of process – in being able to see a practice like community work as comprising a range of tasks that can be placed in a sequence that has a beginning, a middle and an ending. The community work process consists of a series of phases, or steps, or stages, or activities. Each phase has its own tasks that need to be carried out both by the worker and the group. In order to carry out these tasks, the participants need to have or acquire certain kinds of knowledge, skills and technologies. For example, in order to carry out the task of analysing census data, the worker and residents need to *know* where to get the census information and what data they need to cull from it; to be *skilled* in analysing, interpreting and presenting this data; and to be able to master some basic *technologies* in doing this work, such as the use of a pocket calculator.

The accomplishment of the tasks at each phase of the process will largely be determined by the effectiveness of the tactics and strategies used by the worker and/or the group to carry out the tasks. It will also be affected by the resources at the disposal of the worker and the group, and also by the style, values, commitment, experience and training of the worker, and by the kind of *role* the worker chooses or is forced to play in the group. The means to accomplishing tasks, and particularly the choice of tactics and strategies, will also be influenced by the opportunities and constraints present in the worker's employing agency.

Perhaps it would be helpful to present two examples of the community work process (more examples will be discussed later in the chapter). The first is that provided by Batten (1967) and illustrates (Figure 11.1) the 'stages through which the members of a group may move from a passive state of feeling only vaguely dissatisfied to some positive action designed to meet some specific want'.

The second example is taken from Brager and Specht (1973) (Table 11.1). Their model of process is based on the four group functions of socialisation, developing affective relationships, organisation building and mediating relationships between people and institutions. Like the Batten model, it indicates the tasks of the community worker at each stage of the process.

These two examples of the community work process are particularly helpful because they illustrate a number of issues about the notion of process. First, they show that the basis for describing the stages of the process will vary from person to person. Batten's stages are constructed upon development in the thinking of the members of a group, whereas Brager and Specht construct their stages on the basis of group functions and development. Second, process models will vary in the number of stages, and in the degree of specificity and abstraction with which the stages and the worker's tasks are described. Third, there are different ways of analysing and describing the tasks of the worker.

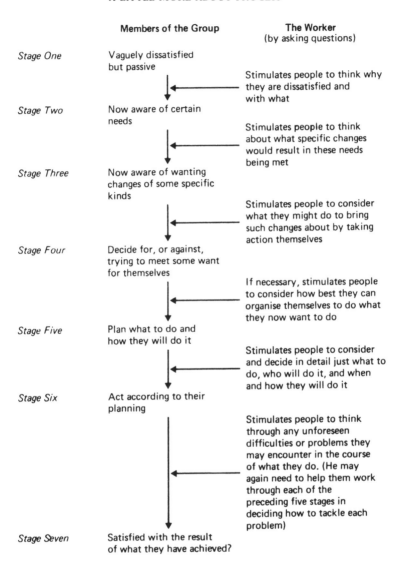

Figure 11.1 *Stages in the thinking process leading to action by a group*

Table 11.1 *Process and tasks in community organisation*

Stages of process	Worker tasks	
	Technical tasks	Interactional tasks
Socialisation groups: socialisation	Identify and define problems	Identify potential members; motivate and recruit members; educate constituency
Primary groups: develop affective relations	Link problem identification to goal development	Cultivate social bonds and build group cohesion
Organisation-development groups: build organisations	Develop programme objectives and organisation structures	Broaden constituency; build a coalition; develop leadership
Institutional relations organisations: mediate in the relations between individuals and institutions	Implement strategy (administration and planning)	Participate in organisational enrichment and change through use of tactics: education, persuasion, bargaining and pressure

Batten's descriptions of these tasks, for example, are largely determined by his idea of the worker's role ('non-directive') whereas Brager and Specht analyse the tasks according to whether they are technical or interactional (and thus implicitly give more emphasis to the knowlege and skill of the worker in carrying out these different kinds of tasks). These differences illustrate the range of process models to be found in the community work literature.

Know-Why Propositions

These are more abstract and, on the whole, are eclectically brought into and used in community work from various academic disciplines, politics and other professions. For example, knowledge from the social sciences, group dynamics or political theories are employed in order better to understand, and hopefully to change, the issues, problems and systems with which the community worker is involved. Kramer and Specht define know-why propositions as 'foundation knowledge about the structure and function of social systems and processes. They include descriptions, explanations, and predictions about how social systems operate under various conditions' (1975).

In brief, the work of know-why propositions is to help workers describe and explain why people, groups, organisations and processes in their environment are functioning as they are; and why issues and problems are arising, persisting and presenting themselves in the way that they are. The purpose of these propositions is to inform the worker's 'know-how' propositions; they are one of the handmaidens of change and workers will rightly accept and reject know-why propositions according to whether or not they aid the doing of community work.

Many books on the teaching of community work discuss the provenance and usefulness of know-why propositions. The ACW book on skills, for example, analyses the contributions of sociology, social psychology, social history, political science, social policy and social administration (1975). There is within each of these and other disciplines a range of schools, camps, positions and orthodoxies from which the community worker can choose and develop know-why propositions. The challenge to any community work trainer is to introduce the material from these disciplines in a 'non-academic' way, alerting the student to its relevance to the practice of community work. Such material is at its most useful to the community worker when she appreciates its integration with 'know-how' propositions.

Know-About Propositions

These kinds of propositions constitute 'knowledge about' community work. Community work itself becomes a focus of study, about which people will develop views, propositions, speculations, theories and even predictions. Propositions that perpetuate knowledge about community work seek to define and understand it as a social, professional and political phenomenon. Such propositions are concerned to locate community work, to describe its situation or place in society, and to delineate the contexts or environments in which it operates and which it may seek to change.

Community workers are not reluctant to engage in discussions *about* community work. How many conferences have we attended, how many papers have we read with titles such as 'Whither community work?', 'Community work: social change or social control?', 'What future community development?', 'Community work: social change or short change?'. One way to understand the predominance of such discussions in British community work is to see them as a development in the growth of a relatively new activity. They are to do with the testing and establishment of a culture with its norms, goals, interests and disputes about affiliation and membership.

'Know-about' propositions and discussion in community work are largely concerned with the following matters:

(1) the function, goals and purposes of community work in society;
(2) the values, assumptions, motivations and ideologies of community work and its practitioners;
(3) the funding, sponsorship and organisational bases for community work;
(4) the relationship of community work to other professions or movements, and the contribution it has made, or is to make, to them;
(5) facilities and procedures available for the training and support of community workers;
(6) categories or typologies of community work; for example, the distinction between neighbourhood work, community organisation and social planning;
(7) process and product in community work, and the kind of balance between the two that is desirable and achievable;
(8) the history and development of community work.

We view the interaction of these various kinds of propositions as highly desirable. It is essential in community work that practitioners are able to hook on to their day-to-day practice both ideas that try to interpret and explain social structures and processes, and discussions about the history, goals and basic assumptions of community work.

We have taken some time to discuss these different kinds of knowledge and propositions in order to safeguard ourselves. This book has been concerned only with the development of a process of neighbourhood work that specifies and orders 'know-how' propositions. We have not discussed the second aspect of practice theory – 'know-why' propositions – nor did we give much attention to matters such as the goals, functions and values of community work. We consider such matters to be of central importance in neighbourhood work, and the reader should not take their absence from this book as any indication that we regard them as trivial or side issues. Our purpose in writing this book was to describe a process account of the tasks and skills in doing neighbourhood work, and we have confined ourselves to this demanding purpose in the face of many temptations to wheel in the 'big issues' around in community work.

We should also point out that in dealing with the process of neighbourhood work we confined ourselves mainly to a discussion of the tasks, roles and skills of the worker. We did not enter into extended discussion about some of the substantive issues currently involved in the practice of neighbourhood work, except in so far as these issues illustrated aspects of practice theory. For example, readers may have been disappointed that we gave insufficient consideraton to issues such as the participation of ethnic groups and women in neighbourhood work; or the relationship of neighbourhood groups to trade unions and trade councils. These matters and others are of clear significance in neighbourhood work and if we neglected in this book to give them a thorough discussion it was only to give ourselves adequate opportunity to develop our account of neighbourhood work as a process.

Process Models in Related Fields

The development of process models in community work has taken place alongside, and been influenced by, the use of process accounts in describing the activities of practitioners in related fields. We shall now briefly indicate the use of process accounts in social work, research, planning and adult education, not only to provide some context for our previous discussion of process in neighbourhood work but also because many of these process accounts are of value for the better carrying-out of some of the activities of neighbourhood work.

Social Work

There are several kinds of process model to be found in the literature on casework and group work. In casework, the traditional process model has been that of diagnosis–treatment–termination and evaluation. Whittaker has elaborated on this basic model, and produced eight phases of the social treatment sequence (1974).

As far as group work is concerned, McCaughan has described a process model for group work practice that is based on the kinds of tasks a worker has to attend to in the different phases of group development (1977a). McCaughan's account of process in group work is of direct usefulness to community workers in thinking about their tasks in relation to the action groups with whom they work.

There are two other sorts of process model to be found in social work practice, and both are rather different from the therapy- or treatment-oriented models. First, there is the 'planned change' model of process in social work, as presented by Lippet, Watson and Westley (1958). They present seven phases in the change process:

(1) development of a need for change;
(2) establishment of a change relationship;
(3) clarification or diagnosis of the client system's problem;
(4) examination of alternative routes and goals; establishing goals and intention of action;
(5) transformation of intentions into actual change efforts;
(6) generalisation and stabilisation of change;
(7) achievement of a terminal relationship.

Lippet, Watson and Westley suggest that changes in persons, groups, organisations and communities can be conceived as comprising this sequences of phases. This process model is both more abstract than those we have previously discussed and less illuminating in this outline form about the specific tasks of the worker or the change-agent. This model is also generic in that it can be used to understand the process of change in a variety of different-sized systems ranging from the individual to the community.

320

The second model of process is equally generic and unitary. It is that offered by Pincus and Minahan as a way of conceptualising the essential practice skills in casework, group work and community work. They identify the following elements of the process of social work practice:

(1) assessing problems;
(2) collecting data;
(3) making initial contacts;
(4) negotiating contracts;
(5) forming action systems;
(6) maintaining and co-ordinating action systems;
(7) exercising influence;
(8) terminating the change effort. (1973)

Pincus and Minahan offer a detailed discussion of the tasks of the worker in each of these eight activities or phases. For example, assessing problems comprises identifying and stating the problem; analysing the dynamics of the social situation; establishing goals and targets; determining tasks and strategies; and stabilising the change effort. They also offer a discussion of *method* at each phase. For example, they discuss questioning, observation and the use of existing written material as methods within the general activity of collecting data.

The models of process developed in casework, group work and unitary approaches to social work practice are of relevance to community work. First, such process accounts have provided a model for the development of ideas of process in community work. Second, they are useful in themselves for furthering thinking about and practice in some of the phases of community work. Third, they indicate that the stages of the work process may be described in either group-centred or worker-centred terms. That is, the stages of the process may be described either in terms of the phases of the growth and development of the group, or in terms of the tasks and skills of the practitioner. Some models, such as that of Brager and Specht referred to earlier, attempt to combine both approaches.

Research

We have chosen to discuss the research process because, first, it is a paradigm of activity based on the careful sequencing and interdependence of a series of tasks; and, secondly, it is useful to community workers in considering the demands made on them in some aspects of the community work process. For example, elements of the research process are clearly pertinent to the community worker's involvement in data collection and needs assessment and in evaluating the effectiveness of his work. The major aspects of the research process comprise the selection of topic for research; problem formulation; research design; data collection; data analysis; the presentation of findings; and the presentation of conclusions and interpretations. Each of these stages of the research process consists of a number of technical, interactional and administrative tasks.

Tripodi has presented a problem-solving model of research that he suggests is analogous to problem-solving models of the 'work conducted by social caseworkers, group workers, community organisers, administrators and policy developers' (1974). Tripodi sees value in establishing this practice–research analogy in order to increase the likelihood of practitioners seeing social research methods as potentially useful in their practice.

Planning

Process models are common to both physical and social planning. Lichfield *et al.* (1975) have developed a detailed process model for physical planning activities. Within social planning, there are several models of the planning process. For instance, that of Kahn (1969) emphasises the technical aspects of planning, while that of Perlman and Gurin (1972) give equal prominence to the interactional or organising tasks of the social planner. We present below a planning process that we have developed in our own teaching:

(1) value exploration and orientation;
(2) preliminary identification and definition of problem areas;
(3) decision to act and definition of the tasks to be carried out, and by whom;
(4) assessment of needs and resources for a specified territory and/or group;
(5) definition of goals and targets;

(6) deciding on priorities among goals;
(7) designing a programme of services and interventions;
(8) mobilising resources, especially finance and support;
(9) implementation and delivery of the programme;
(10) evaluation.

We have not built in interactional tasks such as fostering staff and community participation as explicit stages in the process, but we see such tasks as relevant to the major stages as outlined above.

Models of process from the planning field have a twofold value for the community worker. First, they draw attention to the need for community workers to become more familiar with the technical aspects of their work. Second, they suggest the kinds of activity, and their related areas of knowledge and skill, in which community workers must engage if they are to achieve change in organisations and influence their policies and plans. Involvement in social planning and policy development offers the *practice* link between neighbourhood work and regional and national issues. (For a further discussion of this issue, see Thomas, 1978b.)

Adult Education

Our final example of a process model comes from adult education. It is the design for learning devised by Knowles (1972). His process design contains the following seven elements:

(1) setting the physical and psychological climate;
(2) mutual planning;
(3) diagnosing needs;
(4) formulating programme objectives;
(5) planning a sequential design of learning activities;
(6) conducting the learning experiences;
(7) evaluating the learning.

Knowles sees adult education as a process of mutual, self-directed inquiry, and his description of the role of the teacher is analogous to that of the community worker: 'They concern themselves ... with preparing and marshalling resources for engaging learners in inquiry according to *process design*, and they

323

define their role as facilitators and resources in the process of inquiry.'

The process of helping adults to learn, and the techniques and philosophies of those involved in community education in Britain and the Third World, are of interest to community workers. Educational or 'process' goals are a central part of community work practice, whether these goals are conceived of as enhancing the civic, group and interpersonal capacities of individuals, or of increasing their political awareness and competence.

Process Models in Community Work

One way of analysing the treatment of process as a framework of intervention which can be broken down into several parts is to make use of two categories: accounts and models of process developed purposefully, and less explicit processes which can be identified in reports and case studies of community work projects. The first tend to be the work of teachers and writers, the second of practitioners, but the division is far from firm. The difference is between process laid out in conceptual terms as a way of describing neighbourhood work, and process lying within accounts of practice situations. The former usually requires interpretation by the student of neighbourhood work, the latter has to be extracted from particular contexts. They are equally relevant to a review of the neighbourhood work process. In the literature, models of the first type have almost exclusively been the product of United States theoreticians, though Batten is a noted exception; and models of the second type, those implicit in accounts of practice, are those most commonly found in descriptions of British practice. As we shall discuss, the predominance of models of the second type in Britain is partly a function of the importance attached to local work, and an emphasis on the setting and activities of the group, rather than on the tasks and roles of the worker.

Accounts of process in community work seem to fall into four broad categories: those influenced by social work, those by community development, those by social planning and those by community action. These distinctions are not easy to make; although social work, community development, social planning and community action differ on several important dimensions, they also share much in common by way of goals, theories and methods of intervention. A further difficulty is the uncertainty and the elasticity of meaning of these four phrases. Our use of them ought thus to be treated critically and heuristically by the reader; we intend to use them only to indicate certain broad differences in the way accounts of process in neighbourhood work have been developed.

Process accounts in the first category have been influenced by social work, and in particular by casework. In America, they are the descriptions of process offered by writers like McClenahan (1922), Pray (1948), Newstetter (1948) and Kraus (1948). In Britain, the social work flavour of the process of community work is to be found in an early article by Roche (1971). It is of significance that the 'social work accounts' are mostly to be found in the early history of community work in this country and America. They represent the initial development of community work as the third partner in the triangle with casework and group work, concerning itself largely with welfare-type issues relating to individuals and families. The emergence in more recent years of other types of process account (discussed below) reflects a considerable widening in the range of issues and agencies with which community work has been concerned.

The characteristics of these accounts of process are based, as Austin and Betten have written about McClenahan, 'on the study–diagnosis–treatment model basic to both social casework and medical practice ... Like studying a family, the organiser must investigate the spirit, temper and point of view held by various sectors of the community' (1977). There is, too, often an explicit interest in the contribution of community work in improving interpersonal and inter-group relations rather than environmental or social structural conditions, and an appreciation of the gains to individual functioning that come from involvement in community activities.

A concern with the competencies of individuals also charac- terises the second kind of process accounts, though here the vocabulary of concern is that of civic competence, group and leadership skills and the capacity to serve others. These are the accounts of community work that developed within, and were influenced by, community development. These accounts of process emphasise the role of the worker coming in from outside to a strange community or country. There is a strong interest in helping local people to become aware and expressive of their needs; to develop programmes and services to meet those needs; and to use resources that are largely to be found within the local communities themselves.

Among the first of these kinds of account is Lindeman's ten steps. They are consciousness of need; spreading the consciousness of need; projection of the consciousness of need; emotional impulse to meet the need quickly; presentation of other solutions; conflict of solutions; investigation; open discussion of issue; integration of solutions; and compromise on the basis of tentative progress (1921).

Two more recent accounts of process within this 'tradition' are those of Batten and the Biddles. The seven-stage process of Batten, in which a group moves from a passive state of dissatisfaction to some positive action, was described earlier in this chapter. The Biddles offer six major stages comprising exploration, organisational, discussional, action, new projects and continuation (1965).

It was probably Arthur Dunham's conception of the stages of community work that marked the first significant appearance of accounts of community work that are influenced by the ideas and language of social planning and social welfare policy. Dunham's problem-solving process comprised the nine steps of recognition of a problem or need; analysis of the problem; fact-finding; planning; official approval; action; recording and reporting; adjustments and evaluation (1958). The emergence of this different way of seeing and describing community work can also be discerned in the book by Leaper which appeared in 1968. And, of course, the first Gulbenkian report that appeared in that year drew attention to the importance of social planning as a strand of community work. The Gulbenkian discussion was heavily influenced by the thinking of Perlman and Gurin, whose book appeared in 1972 but was in fact available in an earlier version to the Gulbenkian group. Later accounts of community work in this mould represent elaborations and refinements of Dunham's process. Amongst the most useful are those of Brager and Specht (1973) (referred to earlier in this chapter), Perlman and Gurin (1972), Spergel (1969), and Schler (1970), whose description of the process of community work represents an integration of the 'community development' and 'social planning' influences on model-building in community work.

These accounts of process in community work were influenced by ideas and developments in the field of territorial and social planning. They indicate an awareness of the technical and analytic components of interventions, and attach at least equal significance to these components in community work as to its interactional or socio-emotional elements. They attempt to bring to community work the expertise, technologies and comprehensiveness of rationalist approaches to planning. In so doing, they try to link local or neighbourhood problems to wider social, political and economic issues, and represent an attempt in community work to engage in organisational, city-wide and regional change.

This is hardly surprising because in the United States such conceptions of the process and practice of community work were born of the hopes for various urban poverty programmes to tackle major social problems in the 1960s. The 'social planning' accounts of the process of community work provide a greater sense of programmatic activity that is in contrast with the fragmented, neighbourhood-centred, individual-centred ethos of other accounts of process in community work, particularly those in the United Kingdom. These 'social planning' acccounts are also suggestive of staff other than community workers being employed on these programmes and initiatives – staff with expertise as planners and as specialists in the problem area that the particular programmes are concerned with.

The fourth 'tradition' of descriptions of the steps in community work is that which we have diffidently called 'community action'. This tradition accounts for most of the attempts by British community workers and teachers to describe the community work process, and they are mostly descriptions of the type that are implicit in literature about projects and individual pieces of work. However, this 'tradition' is one firmly rooted in the writings of two Americans, Saul Alinsky (especially *Rules for Radicals*, 1971), and Warren Haggstrom (1969).

The extent to which a sense of process is made more explicit varies from author to author. In describing the work of the Southwark Community Project, Thomas suggests a process of establishing an organisation; identifying those who make decisions about resources; developing skills and confidence within a group;

and negotiating with those who make decisions about resources (1976). Likewise, the account by Taylor *et al.* (1976) of a Young Volunteer Force Foundation project and by Barr (1977) of neighbourhood work done in the Oldham CDP suggest several distintive phases of community work. Less explicit notions of process are the descriptions of community work in Glasgow by Jacobs (1976) and in Notting Hill by O'Malley (1977), though she does refer explicitly to the influence of Richard Hauser's idea of process.

The major force of the 'community action' tradition is neighbourhood work as 'local struggles', and there is a powerful 'political' flavour to this work. The meanings of this term 'political' include both an attempt to relate local issues and problems to social structural factors, and an interest in fostering increased political awareness among local people who take part in neighbourhood action. The relation of local issues to national and international factors is seen as a political matter and not a technical one, as in the 'social planning' tradition.

The process of community work − or more specifically neighbourhood work − in this tradition lies implicit in most accounts partly because of a distrust of 'theorising' that has been felt by many workers in community action, and partly because of a related suspicion of 'professionalism'. This latter suspicion leads workers to 'demystify' the process and nature of neighbourhood work and to present 'ordinary language' descriptions of their work; these descriptions are often written more as contributions to the history of working-class struggles at the neighbourhood level than as guides to a future generation of community workers whose interest in learning 'know-how' propositions would suggest the need for a more explicitly processual account of community work.

The process accounts of the community action tradition share with those more influenced by community development a concern with identifying and raising awareness about local needs and issues. An important difference, however, is that local people are not perceived as objects or recipients of community work inputs and other services; there is a sense in this tradition of collaborative endeavour, with local people being seen as co-campaigners, equal and leading participants in the process of neighbourhood change.

We have already suggested caution in the use of the four

'traditions' of process that we have described above. We hope they serve to indicate the varied ways in which the steps or phases of community work may be sequenced and described. There are, however, a few other qualifying remarks that we wish to make. First, all four 'traditions' offer process accounts that should be treated largely as generic, of use to workers in a variety of agencies and roles. It is not our wish to suggest, for instance, that a worker in a social work agency should, or can only, use a processs account of community work associated with the 'social work tradition'. On the contrary, workers should choose that particular model to conceptualise their work that has the most explanatory and prescriptive power for the circumstances in which they are placed. Spergel (1969) has made this point clear in his discussion of role in community work. His 'social planning' model of the steps of community work comprises problem identification; study; analysis; goal development; planning; intervention; evaluation and feed-back. The ordering of work in these phases is pertinent whether the practitioner sees his or her role as enabler, advocate, organiser or developer.

It is not required of community workers who want to use process accounts of the social planning kind that they are skilled or knowledgeable in planning techniques and ideas, nor that they share any ideological or professional assumptions which they think inherent in such accounts. A community activist may be attracted to a social-planning-type model because it helps to make sense of the turbulent action in which the worker and others are engaged. Recognition that process models differ raises the issue of *choice*: on what basis does the community worker choose which process model to use in conceptualising and guiding his work? None of the models that we have discussed is more 'right' or 'correct' than any of of the others, and the worker's choice will be guided by his own values, intellectual predispositions, and the degree to which he has found particular models *helpful* in understanding and improving his practice.

The particular value of most of the process accounts in all four 'traditions' is twofold. First, they attempt to be comprehensive and thorough. They attempt to disaggregate the process of community work into workable and meaningful steps, on each of which there are a variety of tasks to be carried out. We may disagree with the description of the steps, and the way in which they are sequenced and the languge in which they are described; we may want to add to or subtract from the number of phases in any given model. But the important factor is that we learn the lesson from them of the value of comprehensive and thorough disaggregation; in being able to differentiate events, people and processes 'out there' in the neighbourhood.

The value of this disaggregation and ordering is largely analytic or intellectual; we do not suggest that what is happening out there is as neatly tied and labelled as in our process accounts, nor that any worker should attempt to force what is happening out there to conform with the phases of the model he or she is using. Rather, it is the models that need to be changed as we test them out against events in practice; a good account of the process of community work is, in effect, one that lends itself to change and adaptation to meet the demands of different practice situations and workers.

A second value is that most process accounts build in phases and periods of reflection and planning. The activities of standing back, taking stock, the exploration of the consequences of alternative courses of action and the thoughtful anticipation of events to come are valued in several models; in community work they are to be valued as safeguards against unthinking activism (in the sense used by Freire) and ensnarement in what Poulton (1980) has called the 'action trap' – taking on more work and commitments at a neighbourhood level than individual or project resources can handle, with a consequent neglect of other responsibilities.

Skill and Craft

The process account which we have offered in this book is a tool, but inevitably it is not neutral – a point made by Boston in a commentary on the work of Freire:

> All too often we tend to regard education as the public transmission of neutral bits of information about the world, which can then be used according to the private disposition of the learner. We regard the material as empty of ideological content, similar to a shovel or a pencil. But even the simplest implements of culture reflect an ideology for Freire. (1975)

One has only to recall the use made by National Front organisers of community work methods for recruiting in parts of London's East End to realise how knowledge and skill can be abused. Writers who strive to assemble valid material for practice theory which can have a broad applicability place themselves on a knife edge. On the one hand they can appear to have no ideology or value system, on the other their work can be misused. The vital safety mechanism lies in the certainty that no author can hope to conceal his convictions and values entirely, however committed he is towards 'objective', broad-based literature. We think there is ample evidence in this text of our own views about neighbourhood work and its relationship to society, despite our wish not to weave politically committed writing into the book.

In training an apprentice to be a locksmith the teacher can have no guarantee that the student will not misuse what he learns. The same is true of neighbourhood work practice theory. What is possible is for the student or reader to be aware of the teacher's or author's value system which underpins the practice theory.

Yet there are other anxieties frequently expressed by neighbourhood workers about learning skills in addition to those of their possible misuse or their masking of values and ideology:

(1) Fear of de-skilling is voiced sometimes because of the possible effect of study and training on the spontaneous, intuitive grasp of some neighbourhood workers in their work with local people.
(2) Identifying a range of skills can be off-putting because this sugegsts that workers need to be competent in all or most of them.
(3) It can be hard for a worker to be aware that he knows he has in fact acquired skills. Again, this reflects the unpredictable, volatile nature of neighbourhood work; no campaign or project will provide blueprints for others. But it is also an expression of the philosophical difficulty of providing comprehensive explanations of 'know-how' propositions: few people can state precisely when they acquired a skill.

This problem was captured for one of the authors during a meeting between himself, a fieldwork supervisor and a student. When commenting on the ability of the student to help organise a public meeting the supervisor exclaimed: 'I don't know how I am sure that someone is skilled at organising a meeting. Learning to do it may take weeks or it may take years. But suddenly I know that it is there, I have no doubts.'

The pull between skill development and intuition is important for neighbourhood work. Spontaneity and creativity, which link closely to intuition, can appear sometimes to be the only resource or strength bringing or holding a group together. That is why, in the introduction to the book, we warned against the dominance of intuition and charisma in neighbourhood work. Yet in working through the different phases of the neighbourhood work process we are aware that this aspect may have become obscured. Often people link it with strong personalities or charismatic leadership but this is to underplay and to distort the significance of intuitive behaviour in neighbourhood work.

Sometimes the sense of the worker that he or she has to respond to demands and priorities which arise becomes very powerful; quite literally, pressures of time necessitate intuitive action. John Edginton's observation that detached youth work requires 'experienced instinct' in its approach to people and events 'rather than any carefully conceived and applied theory of practice' (1979) is appropriate also for neighbourhood work.

When we use material on neighbourhood work skills in training workshops the need for reflex action is demonstrated: for example, workers use role plays and video to practise making contact with local people in a south London betting shop, a working men's club on a Yorkshire council estate or a community centre in an Oxfordshire village. We find that such situations must bring into play the natural, instinctive moves of any neighbourhood worker. You cannot learn everything, you perform it – possibly because you have done it many times before, in tiny different ways. The following description by Gibson of the neighbourhood worker's reaction to the verbal demand by a tough group of Scottish teenagers to the director of social work for a share in future facilities on a council estate helps convey what we mean:

> He [the director] handed them straight over to the newly appointed neighbourhood worker, Ralph Ibbott, who put the question back to them: will you tell us what you want? Yes,

332

they would, but there must be time and place provided to do it properly. He stepped across the floor, then and there, to the Tenants' Association Chairperson and got her, possibly before she quite realised what was happening, to offer these notorious knife-carrying youngsters the use of the Association's hut in a few days' time. The group turned up on schedule, met Ralph Ibbott and Danny Keenan (whose work with the 10–12 year olds had first caught their fancy) and told them what was what. (1979)

One consequence of drawing attention to what could be called the craft element in neighbourhood work is to retain the tentative character of the skills which have been discussed. The reader will have noted that on several occasions we refer to a skill being useful at more than one stage in the neighbourhood work process. We have also often indicated how the action of a worker will depend to a great extent on his or her own predisposition – whether, for example, a worker favours a more directive or non-directive approach. One is aware too of how the various stages of the process overlap and inter-relate with each other, especially how early on study and planning do merge into action. For all these reasons we have refrained from attempting to categorise the skills under examination or to draw up a list.

Bibliography

Abrams, M. (1951), *Social Surveys and Social Action* (London: Heinemann).

Adamson, J., and Warren, C. (1983), *Welcome to St Gabriel's Family Centre* (London: Children's Society).

Algie, J., Miller, C. and Kam, N. (1977), 'Management, planning and community work', in *Community Work: Learning and Supervision*, ed. C. Briscoe and D. Thomas (London: Allen & Unwin).

Alinsky, S. (1969), *Reveille for Radicals* (New York: Vintage Books).

Alinsky, S. (1971), *Rules for Radicals* (New York: Random House).

Archbishop of Canterbury's Commission on Urban Priority Areas (1985), *Faith in the City: A Call for Action by Church and Nation* (London: Church House Publishing).

Armstrong, J. and Key, M. (1979), 'Evaluation, change and community work', *Community Development Journal*, vol. 14, no. 3 (October).

Arnstein, S. (1969), 'A ladder of citizen participation', *Journal of American Institute of Planners*, vol. 35, no. 4 (July).

Association of Community Workers (1975), *Knowledge and Skills for Community Work* (London: ACW).

ACW (1978), *Conditions of Employment for those Working in the Community* (London: ACW).

ACW (1979), *The Community Workers' Skills Manual* (London: ACW).

Astin, B. (1979), 'Linking an information centre to community development', in *Collective Action*, ed. M. Dungate, P. Henderson and L. Smith (London: CPF/ACW).

Austin, M. J. and Betten, N. (1977), 'Intellectual origins of community organising, 1920–1939', *Social Service Review*, March.

Bailey, R. (1973), *The Squatters* (Harmondsworth: Penguin).

Baldock, P. (1974), *Community Work and Social Work* (London: Routledge & Kegan Paul).

Baldock, P. (1977), 'The community worker's group and training', in *Community Work: Learning and Supervision* ed. C. Briscoe and D. Thomas (London: Allen & Unwin).

Barclay Report (1982), *Social Workers; Their Role and Tasks* (London: Bedford Square Press).

Barr, A. (1977), *The Practice of Neighbourhood Community Work* (York: Department of Social Administration and Social Work).

Batten, T. R. (1967), *The Non-Directive Approach in Group and Community Work* (Oxford: OUP).

Benington, J. (1975), 'Gosford Green residents' association: a case study', in *The Sociology of Community Action*, ed. P. Leonard (Keele: University of Keele).

Benwell Community Project (1978), *The Making of a Ruling Class* (Newcastle: Benwell Community Project).

Beynon, H. (1975), *Working for Ford* (Wakefield: E. P. Publishing).

Biddle, W. W., and Biddle, L. J. (1965), *The Community Development Process* (New York: Holt, Rinehart & Winston).

Biddle, W. W., and Biddle, L. J. (1968), *Encouraging Community Development* (New York: Holt, Rinehart & Winston).

Bogdan, R., and Taylor, S. J. (1975), *Introduction to Qualitative Research Methods* (New York: Wiley).

Bond, N. (1975), 'The Hillfields information centre: a case study', in *Action-Research in Community Development*, ed. R. Lees and G. Smith (London: Routledge & Kegan Paul).

Boston, B. O. (1975), 'Paulo Freire: notes of a loving critic', in *Conscientization* (Geneva: Commission on the Churches' Participation in Development).

Brager, G., and Specht, H. (1969), 'Mobilising the poor for social action', in *Readings in Community Organisation* (1st edn), ed. R. Kramer and H. Specht (Englewood Cliffs, NJ: Prentice-Hall).

Brager, G., and Specht, H. (1973), *Community Organising* (New York: Columbia University Press).

Briscoe, C. (1977), 'The consultant in community work', in *Learning and Supervision in Community Work*, ed. C. Briscoe and D. Thomas (London: Allen & Unwin).

Bryant, R. (1974), 'Linking community and industrial action', *Community Development Journal*, vol. 9, no. 1. (January).

Bryant, B. and Bryant, R. (1982), *Change and Conflict: A Study of Community Work in Glasgow* (Aberdeen: Aberdeen University Press).

Bryant, R., and Holmes, B. (1977), 'Fieldwork teaching', in *Community Work: Learning and Supervision*, ed. C. Briscoe and D. Thomas (London: Allen & Unwin).

Burghardt, S. (1977), 'A community organisation typology of group development', *Journal of Sociology and Welfare*, vol. IV, no. 7 (September).

Butcher, H. (1976), 'Neighbourhood information centres – access or advocacy?', *Journal of Social Policy*, vol. 5, no. 4 (October).

Butcher, H., *et al.* (1980), *Community Groups in Action: Case Studies and Analysis* (London: Routledge & Kegan Paul).

Calouste Gulbenkian Foundation (1984), *A National Centre for Community Development* (London: CGF).

Cambridge General Improvement Areas (1978), 'Information note 2', mimeo.

Cartwright, J. (1973), 'Problems, solutions and strategies: a contribution to the theory and practice of planning', *Journal of the American Institute of Planners*, vol. 39, no. 3 (May); also in *Planning for Social Welfare*, ed. N. Gilbert and H. Specht (Englewood Cliffs, NJ: Prentice-Hall, 1977).

Cary, L. J. (1975), 'The role of the citizen in the community development process', in *Community Development as a Process* ed. L. J. Cary (Columbia: University of Missouri).

Central Council for Education and Training in Social Work (1974), *The Teaching of Community Work* (London: CCETSW).

Cheeseman, D., Lansley, J., and Wilson, J. (1972), *Neighbourhood Care and Old People. A Community Development Project* (London: Bedford Square Press).

Cheetham, J., and Hill, M. (1973), 'Community work: social realities and ethical dilemmas', *British Journal of Social Work*, vol. 3, no. 3 (autumn).

City Lit (1978), *Learning Through Local Management* (London: Adult Education Training Unit, The City Lit).

Clarke, S., and Henderson, P. (1978), *Friends Neighbourhood House* (London: Friends Community Relations Comittee).

Cleveland County Social Services Department (1978), *Neighbourhood Work: Brambles Farm Project* (Cleveland: County Social Services Department, Environmental Social Development Section).

Clinard, M. B. (1966), *Slums and Community Development: Experiments in Self-Help* (London: Collier-Macmillan).

Community Action (1974), 'Community organisation', *Community Action*, no. 12 (February–March).

Community Action (1975a), 'How to organise and run public meetings', *Community Action*, no. 19 (April–May).

Community Action (1975b), 'Organising a petition', *Community Action*, no. 20 (June–July).

Community Action (1975c), *Investigator's Handbook* (London: Community Action).

Community Action (1976), 'Membership – getting people involved', *Community Action*, no. 28 (November–December).

Community Action (1978), 'Starting to organise', *Community Action*, no. 39 (September–October).

Community Development Journal (1979), papers for Bristol conference, ACW/NISW, vol. 14, no. 3 (November).

Community Development Project (1974), *Inter-Project Report* (London: CDP).

Community Development Project (1975), *The Forward Plan* (London: CDP).

Community Development Project (1977), *The Costs of Industrial Change* (London: CDP Inter-Project Editorial Team).

Community Projects Foundation (1977), *Community Groups Handbook* (London: CPF).

Cooper, B. M. (1966), *Writing Technical Reports* (Harmondsworth: Pelican).

Corkey, D. (1975), 'Early stages in North Tyneside CDP', in *Action-Research in Community Development*, ed. R. Lees and G. Smith (London: Routledge & Kegan Paul).

Coventry CDP (1975), *Final Report* (Coventry: CDP/Institute of Local Government Studies).

Cowan, J. (1979), 'Starting neighbourhood work on a council estate', in *Collective Action: A Selection of Community Work Case Studies*, ed. M. Dungate, P. Henderson and L. Smith (London: ACW).

Cox, D. (1970), *A Community Approach to Youth Work in East London* (London: YWCA).

Cox, F. M. *et al.* (1977), *Tactics and Techniques of Community Practice* (Itasca, Ill.: Peacock).

Craig, G., *et al.* (1892), *Community Work and the State: Towards a Radical Practice* (London: Routledge & Kegan Paul).

Crossley, R., de Groot, L., and McLean, A. (1977), 'Tenants co-ops', mimeo., available from Holloway Tenant Co-operative.

Darvill, G. (1975), *Bargain or Barricade* (Berkhamsted: The Volunteer Centre).

Davies, C., and Crousaz, D. (1982), *Local Authority Community Work: Realities and Practice* (London: DHSS).

Dearlove, J. (1973), *The Politics of Policy in Local Government* (Cambridge: CUP).

Delbecq, A. L., and Van de Ven, A. H. (1971), 'A group process model for problem identification and program planning', *Journal of Applied Behavioural Science* (September); also in *Planning for Welfare* (1977), ed. N. Gilbert and H. Specht (Englewood Cliffs, NJ: Prentice-Hall).

Dennis, N. (1968), 'The popularity of the neighbourhood community', in *Readings in Urban Sociology*, ed. R. E. Pahl (Oxford: Pergamon).

Dennis, N. (1970), *People and Planning* (London: Faber).

Department of the Environment (1977), *A Voice for your Neighbourhood* (London: HMSO).

Douglass, R. L. (1977), 'How to use and present community data', in *Tactics and Techniques of Community Practice*, ed. F. M. Cox *et al.* (Itasca, Ill.: Peacock).

Dunham, A. (1958), *Community Welfare Organisation: Principles and Practice* (New York: Crowell).

Dunham, A. (1970), *The New Community Organisation* (New York: Crowell).

Dymond, D. (1981), *Writing Local History* (London: Bedford Square Press).

Ecklein, J. L., and Lauffer, A. A. (1972), *Community Organisers and Social Planners* (New York: Wiley).

Edginton, J. (1979), *Avenues Unlimited* (Leicester: National Youth Bureau).

Edwards, J. (1975), 'Social indicators, urban deprivation and positive discrimination', *Journal of Social Policy*, vol. 4 (July).

Epstein, I., *et al.* (1973), 'Community development programmes and their evaluation', *Community Development Journal*, vol. 8 no. 1 (January).

Etzioni, A. (1967), 'Mixed-scanning: a "third" approach to decision-making', *Public Administration Review*, 1 (December); also in N. Gilbert and H. Specht *Planning for Social Welfare* (Englewood Cliffs, NJ: Prentice-Hall, 1977).

Euguster, C. (1974), 'Field education in West Heights: equipping a deprived community to help itself', in *Strategies of Community Organisation*, ed. F. Cox *et al.* (Itasca, Ill.: Peacock).

Family Service Units (1974), 'Community work from day to day', by Jenny Morton, *FSU Quarterly*, no. 7 (summer).

Foster, J. (1975), 'Working with tenants: two case studies', in *Action-Research in Community Development*, ed. R. Lees and G. Smith (London: Routledge & Kegan Paul).

Francis, D., *et al.* (1984). *A Survey of Community Workers in the United Kingdom* (London: National Institute for Social Work).

Freire, P. (1972a), *Cultural Action for Freedom* (Harmondsworth: Penguin).

Freire, P. (1972b), *Pedagogy of the Oppressed* (Harmondsworth: Penguin).

Gallagher, A. (1977), 'Women and community work', in *Women in the Community*, ed. M. Mayo (London: Routledge & Kegan Paul).

Garland, J. A. *et al.* (1972), 'A model for stages of development in social work groups', in *Explorations in Group Work: Essays in Theory and Practice*, ed. S. Bernstein (London: Bookstall Publications).

Gibson, T. (1978), *Neighbourhood Action Packs* (Nottingham: University of Nottingham).

Gibson, T. (1979), *People Power* (Harmondsworth: Penguin).

Gibson, T. (1984), *Counterweight: The Neighbourhood Option* (London: Town and Country Planning Association).

Gilbert, N., and Specht, H. (1974), *Dimensions of Social Welfare Policy* (Englewood Cliffs, NJ: Prentice-Hall).

Gilbert, N., and Specht, H. (1977), *Planning for Social Welfare* (Englewood Cliffs, NJ: Prentice-Hall).

Glampson, A. *et al.* (1975), *A Guide to the Assessment of Community Needs and Resources* (London: NISW).

Glen, A., Pearce, J., and Booth, A. (1977), *Resources for Social Change* (York: Papers in Community Studies, No. 14).

Godrey, W. (1985), *Down to Earth: Stories of Church Based Community Work* (London: British Council of Churches).

Goetschius, G. W. (1969, 1971), *Working with Community Groups* (London: Routledge & Kegan Paul).

Gold, R. L. (1969), 'Roles in sociological field observations', in *Issues in Participant Observation*, ed. G. J. McCall and J. L. Simmons (Reading, Mass.: Addison-Wesley).

Goodenough, E. H. (1963), *Co-operation in Change: An Anthropological Approach to Community Development* (New York: Russell Sage).

Green, G. (1975), 'The leasehold problem in Saltley', in *Action-Research in Community Development*, ed. R. Lees and G. Smith (London: Routledge & Kegan Paul).

Grosser, C. F. (1968), 'Staff role in neighbourhood organisation', in *Neighbourhood Organisation for Community Action*, ed. J. Turner (New York: NASW).

Grosser, C. F. (1975), 'Community development programs serving the urban poor', in *Readings in Community Organisation Practice* (2nd edn), ed. R. Kramer and H. Specht (Englewood Cliffs, NJ: Prentice-Hall).

Gulbenkian Community Work Group (1973), *Current Issues in Community Work* (London: Routledge & Kegan Paul).

Haggstrom, W. C. (1969), 'Can the poor transform the world?' in *Readings in Community Organisation Practice* (1st edn), ed. R. Kramer and H. Specht (Englewood Cliffs, NJ: Prentice-Hall).

Haggstrom, W. C. (1970), 'The psychological implications of the community development process', in *Community Development as a Process*, ed. L. J. Cary (Columbia: University of Missouri Press).

Hampton, W. (1973), *The Neighbourhood and the Future* (London: ACW).

Harris, P. (1977), 'Staff supervision in community work', in *Community Work: Learning and Supervision*, ed. C. Briscoe and D. N. Thomas (London: Allen & Unwin).

Hartford, M. E. (1971), *Groups in Social Work* (New York: Columbia University Press).

Hasenfeld, Y. (1977), 'Analysing the human service agency's interorganisational relations and internal characteristics', in *Tactics and Techniques of Community Practice*, ed. F. M. Cox et al. (Itasca, Ill.: Peacock).

Hatch, S., and Sherrott, R. (1973), 'Positive discrimination and the distribution of deprivations', *Policy and Politics*, vol. 1, no. 3 (March).

Hatch, S., et al. (1977), *Research and Reform: Southwark CDP 1969–1972* (London: Hatch et al.).

Heap, K. (1985), *The Practice of Social Work with Groups* (London: Allen & Unwin).

Hedley, R., et al. (1985), *Your Neighbourhood Group* (London: ADVANCE).

Heeran, R. (1980), 'Professionalism, roles and conflict', mimeo., NISW.

Helier, T. (n.d.), Notes from a GP on the politics of self-help', *Spotlight* (Self-Help Clearing House), no. 5, pp. 9 and 10.

Henderson, P. (1978), *Community Work and the Local Authority* (Manchester: Manchester Monographs 12).

Henderson, P., and Scott, T. (1984), *Learning More about Community Social Work* (London: National Institute for Social Work).

Henderson, P., and Thomas, D. N. (1980), *Readings in Community Work* (London: Allen & Unwin).

Henderson, P., and Thomas, D. N. (1981), 'Federations of community groups – the benefits and dangers', *Community Development Journal* (April).

Henderson, P., et al. (1980), *The Boundaries of Change in Community Work* (London: Allen & Unwin).

Henderson, P., et al. (1983), *Success and Struggles on Council Estates – Tenant Action and Community Work* (London: ACW).

HMSO (1968), *Report of the Committee on Local Authority and Allied Personal Social Services*, Seebohm Report, Cmnd 3703.

Hoinville, G., et al (1978), *Survey Research Practice* (London: Heinemann).

Holman, R. (1983), *Resourceful Friends: Skills in Community Social Work* (London: Children's Society).

Holmes, C. (1977), 'Islington's tough approach works', *Roof*, vol. 2, no. 3 (May).

Honor Oak Estate Neighbourhood Association (1977), *A Street Door of Our Own* (London: Honor Oak Estate Neighbourhood Association).

Hoskins, W. G. (1968), *Local History in England* (London: Longman).

Houlton, B. (1975), *The Activists' Handbook* (London: Arrow).

Huber, L., and McCartney, F. (1980), 'A neighbourhood approach to community work', in *Boundaries of Change in Community Work*, ed. P. Henderson, D. Jones and D. N. Thomas (London: Allen & Unwin).

Inter-Action Advisory Service (1975), *Basic Video in Community Work*, Handbook no. 5 (London: Inter-Action Imprint).

Iredale, D. (1974), *Local History Research and Writing* (Leeds: The Elinfield Press).

Jackson, K. (1970), 'Adult educaiton and community development', *Studies in Adult Education*, vol. 2, no. 2 (November).

Jacobs, J. (1972), *The Death and Life of Great American Cities* (Harmondsworth: Penguin).

Jacobs, S. (1976), *The Right to a Decent House* (London: Routledge & Kegan Paul).

Janes, R. (1969), 'A note on phases of the community role of the participant observer', in *Issues in Participant Observation*, ed. G. J. McCall and J. L. Simmons (Reading, Mass.: Addison-Wesley).

Jordan, B. (1973), *Paupers: The Making of the New Claiming Class* (London: Routledge & Kegan Paul).

Kahn, A. (1969), *Theory and Practice of Social Planning* (New York: Russell Sage).

Kahn, S. (1970), *How People Get Power* (New York: McGraw-Hill).

Key, M., *et) al.* (1976), *Evaluation Theory and Community Work* (London: Young Volunteer Force Foundation).

Khinduka, S. K. (1975), 'Community development: potential and limitations', in *Readings in Community Organisation Practice* (2nd edn), ed. R. Kramer and H. Specht (Englewood Cliffs, NJ: Prentice-Hall).

Knittle, B. (1976), 'The community as client', *International Social Work*, vol. XIX, no. 1.

Knowles, M. (1972), 'Innovations in teaching styles and approaches based on adult learning', *Journal of Education for Social Work*, vol. 8, no. 2, pp. 32–9.

Kramer, R. M. and Specht, H. (1975), *Readings in Community Organisation* (2nd edn) (Englewood Cliffs, NJ: Prentice-Hall).

Kraus, H. (1948), 'Community organisation in social work – a note on choices and steps', *Social Forces* (October).

Lambert, J. (1977), 'Putting things into perspective: research methods and community work', in *Community Work: Learning and Supervision*, ed. C. Briscoe and D. N. Thomas (London: Allen & Unwin).

Lambert, J., and Pearson, J. (1974), *Adventure Playgrounds* (Harmondsworth: Penguin).

League of California Cities (1974), *Assessing Human Needs* (Sacramento: League of California Cities).

Leaper, R. A. B. (1968), *Community Work* (London: NCSS).

Lees, R. (1975), 'You and research: community self survey', *Social Work Today*, vol. 5, no. 22 (6 February).

Leissner, A. (1967), *Family Advice Services* (London: Longman).

Lichfield, N. *et al.* (1975), *Evaluation in the Planning Process* (Oxford: Pergamon).

Lindeman, E. C. (1921), *The Community: An Introduction to the Study of Community Leadership and Organisation* (New York: Association Press).

Lippett, R., *et al.* (1958), *The Dynamics of Planned Change* (New York: Harcourt).

London Neighbourhood Workers' Group (1977), *Newsletter*, no. 13 (LNWG).

Lovett, T. (1975), *Adult Education, Community Development and the Working Class* (London: Ward Lock).

McCall, G. J., and Simmons, J. L. (1969), *Issues in Participant Observation* (Reading, Mass.: Addison-Wesley).

McCaughan, N. (1977a), 'Social group work in the United Kingdom', in *Integrating Social Work Methods*, ed. H. Specht and A. Vickery (London: Allen & Unwin).

McCaughan, N. (1977b), 'Group behaviour: some theories for practice', in *Community Work: Learning and Supervision*, ed. C. Briscoe and D. N. Thomas (London: Allen & Unwin).

McCaughan, N., and Scott, T. (1978), *Role Play and Simulation Games*, National Institute for Social Work Papers, No. 9 (London: NISW).

McClenahan, B. A. (1922), *Organising the Community* (New York: Association Press).

McGrath, M. (1975a), 'Social needs of an immigrant population', in *Action-Research in Community Development*, ed. R. Lees and G. Smith (London: Routledge & Kegan Paul).

McGrath, M. (1975b), 'For the people by the people – a resident run advice centre', *British Journal of Social Work*, vol. 5, no. 3 (autumn).

Mackay, A. (1975), 'Expectations of a local project', in *Action Research in Community Development*, ed. R. Lees and G. Smith (London: Routledge & Kegan Paul).

Mayo, M. (1975), 'The history and early development of CDP', in *Action Research in Community Development*, ed. R. Lees and G. Smith (London: Routledge & Kegan Paul).

Mayo, M. (1977), *Women in the Community* (London: Routledge & Kegan Paul).

Meld, M. B. (1974), 'The politics of evaluation of social programs', *Social Work*, vol. 19, no. 4. (July).

Miller, J. (1979), *Waterloo Health Project 1978–79* (London: Waterloo Action Centre).

Mills, C. W. (1959), *The Sociological Imagination* (New York: OUP).

Mitchell, J. (1974), *How to Write Reports* (London: Fontana).

Mitton, R., and Morrison, E. (1972), *A Community Project in Notting Dale* (London: Allen Lane).

Molnar, D., and Kammerud, M. (1975), 'Problem analysis: the Delphi technique', *Socio-Economic Planning Science*, 9; also in *Planning for Social Welfare*, ed. N. Gilbert and H. Specht (Englewood Cliffs, NJ: Prentice-Hall, 1977).

Moseley, L. G. (1971), 'Evaluative research in community development: a missing dimension', *Community Development Journal*, vol. 6, no. 3 (autumn).

Moser, C. A., and Kalton, G. (1975), *Survey Methods in Social Investigaiton* (2nd edn) (London: Heinemann).

National Council of Social Service (1972), *A Short Guide to Social Survey Methods* (London: Bedford Square Press).

Newman, O. (1972), *Defensible Space* (London: Architectural Press).

Newstetter, W. I. (1948), 'The social intergroup work process', *Proceedings, National Conference of Social Work, 1947* (New York: Columbia University Press).

Newton, K. (1976), *Second City Politics* (Oxford: Clarendon Press).

North Tyneside CDP (1978), 'North Shields: living with industrial change', in *Final Report*, Vol. 2 (Newcastle-upon-Tyne: Newcastle-upon-Tyne Polytechnic).

Northern, H. (1969), *Social Work with Groups* (New York: Columbia University Press).

Norton, M. (1977), *The Directory of Social Change*, Vol. 2 (London: Wildwood House).

O'Brien, D. J. (1975), *Neighbourhood Organisation and Interest Group Processes* (Princeton, NJ: Princeton University Press).

Ohlin, L. E. (1969), 'Urban community development', in *Readings in Community Organisation Practice* (1st edn), ed. R. Kramer and H. Specht (Englewood Cliffs, NJ: Prentice-Hall).

Ohri, A., *et al.* (1982), *Community Work and Racism* (London: Routledge & Kegan Paul).

O'Malley, J. (1977), *The Politics of Community Action* (Nottingham: Spokesman).

Oppenheim, A. N. (1968), *Questionnaire Design and Attitude Measurement* (London: Heinemann).

Palmer, D. (1978), 'Some comments on the problems of tenant involvement', paper for NISW seminar (mimeo.).

Patti, R. J., and Resnick, H. (1975), 'Changing the agency from within', in *Readings in Community Organisation Practice* (2nd edn), ed. R. Kramer and H. Specht (Englewood Cliffs, NJ: Prentice-Hall).

Perlman, R., and Gurin, A. (1972), *Community Organisation and Social Planning* (New York: Wiley).

Perrow, C. (1970), *Organisational Analysis* (London: Tavistock).

Pincus, A., and Minahan, A. (1973), *Social Work Practice: Model and Method* (Itasca, Ill.: Peacock).

Polanshek, K. (1979), 'A city-wide housing action area group', in *Collective Action*, ed. P. Henderson *et al.* (London: CPF/ACW).

Popplestone, G. (1972), 'Collective action among private tenants', *British Journal of Social Work*, vol. 2, no. 3.

Poulton, G. (1980), 'A study in community education' in *Boundaries of Change in Community Work*, ed. P. Henderson, D. Jones and D. N. Thomas (London: Allen & Unwin).

Power, A. (1977), *Five Years On* (London: Holloway Tenant Co-operative).

Pray, K. L. M. (1948), 'When is community organisation social work practice?', *Proceedings, National Conference of Social Work, 1947* (New York: Columbia University Press).

Remfrey, P. (1979), 'North Tyneside Community Development Project', *Community Development Journal*, vol. 14, no. 3 (October).

Rice, A. K. (1965), *Learning for Leadership* (London: Tavistock).

Richardson, A. (1984), *Working with Self-Help Groups* (London: Bedford Square Press).

Robertson, I. (1976), *Community Self-Surveys in Urban Renewal* (Manchester: Manchester Monographs 4).

Roche, E. (1971), 'Guide to community work in seven simple stages', *Social Work Today*, vol. 1, no. 11 (February).

Ross, M. (1967), *Community Organisation* (2nd edn) (London: Harper & Row).

Rothman, J. (1969), 'An analysis of goals and roles in community organisation practice', in *Readings in Community Organisation Practice* (1st edn), ed. R. Kramer and H. Specht (Englewood Cliffs, NJ: Prentice-Hall).

Rothman, J. (1974a), 'Three models of community organisation practice', in *Strategies of Community Organisation* (2nd edn), ed. F. M. Cox *et al.* (Itasca, Ill.: Peacock).

Rothman, J. (1974b), *Planning and Organising for Social Change* (New York: Columbia University Press).

Rothman, J., Erlich, J. L., and Teresa, J. G. (1976), *Promoting Innovation and Change in Organisations and Communities* (New York: Wiley).

Rowbotham, S. (1974), *Woman's Consciousness, Man's World* (Harmondsworth: Penguin).

Rustin, M. (1967–8), 'Community organising in England – Notting Hill Summer Project 1967', *ALTA* (University of Birmingham Review).

Sanders, I. T. (1973), 'The community social profile', in *Perspectives on the American Community*, ed. R. L. Warren (New York: Rand McNally).

Savill, D. (1980), 'Community groups as employers', in *Boundaries of Change in Community Work*, ed. P. Henderson, D. Jones and D. N. Thomas (London: Allen & Unwin).

Schler, D. (1970), 'The community development process', in *Community Development as a Process*, ed. L. J. Cary (Columbia: University of Missouri Press).

Schoenberg, S. P. (1979), 'Criteria for evaluation of neighbourhood vitality in working-class and poor areas in core cities' *Social Problems*, vol. 27, no. 1 (October).

343

Schoenberg, S. P., and Rosenbaum, P. L. (1980), *Neighbourhoods that Work: Sources for Viability in the Inner City* (New Jersey: Rutgers University Press).

Selltiz, C., *et al.* (1976), *Research Methods in Social Relations* (3rd edn) (New York: Holt, Rinehart & Winston).

Shelter Community Action Team (n.d.) *How to Use the Census* (London: Shelter Community Action Team).

Sieder, V. M. (1969), 'Community organisation in the direct-service agency', in *Readings in Community Organisation Practice*, ed. R. Kramer and H. Specht (Englewood Cliffs, NJ: Prentice-Hall).

Smith, G., Lees, R., and Topping, P. (1977), 'Participation and the Home Office community development project in Britain', in *British Political Sociology Yearbook*, ed. C. Crouch (London: Croom Helm).

Smith, L., and Jones, D. (1981), *Deprivation, Participation and Community Action* (London: Routledge & Kegan Paul).

Smythe, P. (1973), 'Action-play', *Community Action*, no. 8 (May–June).

Specht, H. (1975), *Community Development in the UK* (London: ACW).

Specht, H. (1976), *The Community Development Project* (London: NISW).

Spence, D. (1978), 'New towns and their employment problems', paper for ACW conference.

Spergel, I. A. (1969), *Community Problem-Solving: The Delinquency Example* (Chicago: University of Chicago Press).

Spergel, I. A. (1975), 'The role of the community worker', in *Readings in Community Organisation Practice* (2nd edn), ed. R. Kramer and H. Specht (Englewood Cliffs, NJ: Prentice-Hall).

Stein, H. D., and Sarnoff, I. (1964), 'A framework for analysing social work's contribution to the identification and resolution of social problems', *Social Welfare Forum*, Official Proceedings of the National Conference on Social Welfare (New York: Columbia University Press).

Strauss, A., *et al*, (1964), *Psychiatric Ideologies and Institutions* (New York: Free Press).

Tasker, L. J. (1978), 'Class, culture and community work', in *Political Issues and Community Work*, ed. P. Curno (London: Routledge & Kegan Paul).

Taylor, M. (1983), *Inside a Community Project – Bedworth Heath* (London: CPF).

Taylor, M., Kestenbaum, A., and Symons, B. (1976), *Principles and Practice of Community Work in a British Town* (London: Community Projects Foundation).

Tetlow, K. (1979), 'Albany Health Project, progress report' mimeo.

Thomas, D. N. (1975a), 'Chaucer House Tenants' Association: a case study', in *The Sociology of Community Action*, ed. P. Leonard (Keele: University of Keele).

Thomas, D. N. (1975b), 'The community worker as stranger: the effects of housing design', in *Community Work Two*, ed. D. Jones and M. Mayo (London: Routledge & Kegan Paul).

Thomas, D. N. (1976), *Organising for Social Change: A Study in the*

Theory and Practice of Community Work (London: Allen & Unwin).

Thomas, D. N. (1978a), 'Journey into the acting community: experiences of learning and change in community groups', in *Group Work: Learning and Supervision*, ed. N. McCaughan (London: Allen & Unwin).

Thomas, D. N. (1978b), 'Community work, social change and social planning', in *Political Issues and Community Work*, ed. P. Curno (London: Routledge & Kegan Paul).

Thomas, D. N. (1980), 'Research and community work', *Community Development Journal* (January).

Thomas, D. N. (1983a), *The Making of Community Work* (London: Allen & Unwin).

Thomas, D. N. (1983b), *Community Work in the Eighties* (London: National Institute for Social Work).

Thomas, D. N. (1986), *White Bolts, Black Locks – Participation in the Inner City* (London: Allen & Unwin).

Thomas, D. N., and Warburton, R. W. (1977), *Community Workers in a Social Services Department: A Case Study* (London: NISW/PSSC).

Tripodi, T. (1974), *Uses and Abuses of Social Research in Social Work* (New York: Columbia University Press).

Tropman, E. J. (1977), 'Staffing committees and studies', in *Tactics and Techniques for Community Practice*, ed. F. M. Cox *et al.* (Itasca, Ill.: Peacock).

Twelvetrees, A. (1973), *Braunstone Neighbourhood Project. The First Six Years* (Leicester: Leicester FSU).

Twelvetrees, A. (1974), 'Neighbourhood work: a personal view', *FSU Quarterly*, no. 7 (summer).

Twelvetrees, A. (1982), *Community Work* (London: Macmillan).

Von Hoffman, N. (1972), 'Finding and making leaders', abstracted in *Community Organisers and Social Planners*, ed. J. L. Ecklein and A. A. Lauffer (New York: Wiley).

Wallman, S. (1982), *Living in South London* (London: Gower).

Warren, R. B., and Warren, D. I. (1977), *The Neighbourhood Organiser's Handbook* (Notre Dame: University of Notre Dame Press).

Warren, R. L. (1955), *Studying Your Community* (New York: Russell Sage).

Warren, R. L. (1963), *The Community in America* (Chicago: Rand-McNally).

Wates, N. (1976), *The Battle for Tolmers Square* (London: Routledge & Kegan Paul).

Weiner, R. S. P. (1972), *Community Self-Survey: A Do-It-Yourself Guide* (Belfast: Northern Ireland Community Relations Commission).

Whittaker, J. (1974), *Social Treatment* (Chicago: Aldine).

Yang, H. (1966), *Fact-Finding with Rural People* (Rome: Food and Agricultural Organisation).

Zurcher, L. A. (1972), 'Stages of development of neighbourhood action groups: the Topeka example' in *Community Organisation*, ed. I. A. Spergel (London: Sage).

345

Zweig, F. M., and Morris, R. (1975), 'The social planning design guide: process and proposal', in *Readings in Community Organisation Practice* (2nd edn), ed. R. Kramer and H. Specht (Englewood Cliffs, NJ: Prentice-Hall).

The National Institute's own series of Publications about working in Neighbourhoods

Learning more about community social work
Written by a group of practice and management staff at the National Institute, this is a recent account of some of the practice and team aspects of community social work.
Paul Henderson, Tony Scott 1984

A survey of community workers in the United Kingdom
Contains figures on the numbers of community workers in the United Kingdom, their employers, salaries, regions, age, sex, ethnicity, training and other data.
David Francis, Paul Henderson, David N. Thomas 1984

Community work in the eighties
A collection of stimulating articles from a number of experienced trainers and practitioners on the ways in which community work in Britain will develop in the 1980s.
Edited by David N. Thomas 1983

Perspectives on patch
The editors have brought together a number of different experiences and ideas about the decentralisation of social work services.
Edited by Ian Sinclair, David N. Thomas 1983

Community workers in a social services department
A case study that explores some of the major issues that face community workers and their managers in social services departments.
David N. Thomas, R. William Warburton 1977

A guide to the assessment of community needs and resources
One of the most useful publications available for those wishing to assess needs and resources in their neighbourhood. Already in its 5th printing.
Ann Glampson, Tony Scott, David N. Thomas 1975

Community work and the probation service: 8 team reports.
An initial report on the development of community work in the probation service.
Paul Henderson 1986

Index

INDEX